PRENATAL CARE

Reaching Mothers, Reaching Infants

Sarah S. Brown, Editor

Committee to Study Outreach
for Prenatal Care

Division of Health Promotion and
Disease Prevention

INSTITUTE OF MEDICINE

NATIONAL ACADEMY PRESS
Washington, D.C.   1988

NATIONAL ACADEMY PRESS   2101 Constitution Avenue, NW   Washington, DC 20418

NOTICE: The project that is the subject of this report was approved by the Governing Board of the National Research Council, whose members are drawn from the councils of the National Academy of Sciences, the National Academy of Engineering, and the Institute of Medicine. The members of the committee responsible for the report were chosen for their special competences and with regard for appropriate balance.

This report has been reviewed by a group other than the authors according to the procedures approved by a Report Review Committee consisting of members of the National Academy of Sciences, the National Academy of Engineering, and the Institute of Medicine.

The Institute of Medicine was chartered in 1970 by the National Academy of Sciences to enlist distinguished members of the appropriate professions in the examination of policy matters pertaining to the health of the public. In this, the Insititute acts under both the Academy's 1863 congressional charter responsibility to be an adviser to the federal government and its own initiative in identifying issues of medical care, research, and education.

This project has been supported by the Ford Foundation, the Carnegie Corporation of New York, the March of Dimes Birth Defects Foundation, the Rockefeller Foundation, and the Division of Maternal and Child Health within the U.S. Department of Health and Human Services (SPRANS Grant No. MCJ-113852-02-HRSA).

Library of Congress Cataloging-in-Publication Data
Prenatal care : reaching mothers, reaching infants / Sarah S. Brown,
    editor : Committee to Study Outreach for Prenatal Care, Division of
    Health Promotion and Diseases Prevention, Institute of Medicine.
        p.   cm.
    Includes bibliographies and index.
    ISBN 0-309-03892-8
    1. Prenatal care.   2. Women's health services.   I. Brown, Sarah
S.   II. Institute of Medicine (U.S.). Committee to Study Outreach
for Prenatal Care
    [DNLM: 1. Prenatal Care.   WQ 175 P9257]
    RG940.P74 1988
    362.1'982—dc19
    DNLM/DLC   88-28991
    for Library of Congress   CIP

Cover Photograph:
CARRIE BORETZ/ARCHIVE

Printed in the United States of America

Commissioned Papers

VIRGINIA CARTOOF, Cartoof Consulting, Dorchester, Massachusetts

RUTH R. FADEN, Professor, Department of Health Policy and Management, School of Hygiene and Public Health, Johns Hopkins University, Baltimore, Maryland

PAUL T. GIBLIN, Associate Professor, Department of Pediatrics, Children's Hospital, Wayne State University, Detroit, Michigan

ROBERT HALPERN, Faculty, The Erikson Institute for Advanced Study in Child Development, Chicago, Illinois

DANA HUGHES, Senior Health Specialist, Children's Defense Fund, Washington, D.C.

KAY JOHNSON, Senior Health Specialist, Children's Defense Fund, Washington, D.C.

MARGARET MCMANUS, McManus Health Policy, Inc., Washington, D.C.

C. ARDEN MILLER, Professor, Department of Maternal and Child Health, University of North Carolina at Chapel Hill, Chapel Hill, North Carolina

MARYBETH PETSCHEK, Senior Staff Associate, Center for Population and Family Health, Columbia University, New York, New York

PAUL PLACEK, Survey Statistician, Division of Vital Statistics, National Center for Health Statistics, Hyattsville, Maryland

MARILYN POLAND, Associate Professor, Department of Obstetrics and Gynecology, Wayne State University Medical School, Detroit, Michigan

SARA ROSENBAUM, Director, Health Division, Children's Defense Fund, Washington, D.C.

Contributed Paper

LORRAINE KLERMAN, Professor of Public Health, Department of Epidemiology and Public Health, Yale University School of Medicine, New Haven, Connecticut

Acknowledgments

This report represents the collaborative efforts of many individuals and groups, especially the members of the supervising committee, who gave generously of their time and wisdom. Joyce Lashof was an exceedingly effective chairman, helping to engage all of the committee's members in various aspects of the project. Lorraine Klerman, in particular, contributed substantially to the report's development by taking a leadership role in analyzing the materials that now appear in Chapters 3 and 4 and in Appendix A, and Bernard Guyer was especially helpful in drafting Chapter 1. The report also reflects the insights and stimulation provided by a number of commissioned papers, the authors of which appear at the beginning of the report.

The contributions of staff members Amy Fine and Anne Hockett were particularly important. Although neither was able to remain on the study staff for the entire duration of the project, each had a major role in shaping it. Blair Potter, the report editor, was very helpful in her careful attention to countless details of both form and substance, and Linda DePugh managed the immense task of typing this long report with grace and humor.

An important part of the committee's work was its review of numerous programs around the country that are trying to improve use of prenatal care. Thirty-one such programs were studied in detail and are summarized in Appendix A. To help develop the appendix, many program leaders worked closely with the committee and staff; they reviewed numerous drafts, answered endless questions, and seemed to have infinite patience for explaining the "real world" of providing prenatal services. Special thanks go to Richard Aubry, Lawrence Berger, Hannah Boulton, Vicki Breitbart, Jeanne Brooks-Gunn, Elizabeth Campbell, Virginia Cartoof, Joan Christison-Lagay, Deborah Coates, Lyn Headley, Cassandra Jackson, Judith Jones, Muriel Keyes, Athole Lennie, Joan Maxwell, Marie McCormick, Marie Meglen, Katherine Messenger, David Olds, Janet Olszewski, Mary Peoples, Linda Randolph, Jacqueline Scott, Donna Strobino, Lois Wandersman, and Terri Wright.

Many other individuals played important roles in the committee's deliberations by providing information, critical analysis, advice, and reviews of draft materials. Sara Rosenbaum of the Children's Defense Fund and her colleagues Dana Hughes and Kay Johnson were exceptionally helpful and merit immense gratitude. Others who assisted the committee include Robert Ball, Michael Bowling, Jan Chapin, Katherine Darabi, Sara dePersio, Jack Hadley, Ian Hill, Marjorie Horn, Charles Johnson, Sarah Johnson, Susan Kelly, Asta Kenney, Milt Kotelchuck, Mary Grace Kovar, Tom McDonald, Diana Mertens, Arden Miller, Jeanette Miller, Elena Nightingale, Gary Richwald, Anne Rosewater, Jeffrey Taylor, Beverly Toomey, and Louise Warrick. Their assistance is much appreciated.

Funding for the study was provided by the Ford Foundation, the Carnegie Corporation of New York, the March of Dimes Birth Defects Foundation, the Rockefeller Foundation, and the Division of Maternal and Child Health within the U.S. Department of Health and Human Services. The support of these groups is gratefully acknowledged.

SARAH S. BROWN
Study Director

Contents

5

CONCLUSIONS AND RECOMMENDATIONS / 135

APPENDIX

A

SUMMARIES OF THE 31 PROGRAMS STUDIED / 163

APPENDIX

B

PRENATAL CARE OUTREACH:
AN INTERNATIONAL PERSPECTIVE / 210
C. Arden Miller

APPENDIX

C

THE MEDICAL MALPRACTICE
CRISIS AND POOR WOMEN / 229
Sara Rosenbaum and Dana Hughes

INDEX / 245

Summary

In 1985, 76.2 percent of all U.S. infants were born to women who began prenatal care in the first trimester of pregnancy, 18.1 percent to women who delayed care until the second trimester, 4.0 percent to women who obtained care only in the third trimester, and 1.7 percent to mothers who had no prenatal care at all. When vital statistics are analyzed to determine rates of adequate care rather than trimester of onset, a slightly different picture emerges. In 1985, only 68.2 percent of all women obtained adequate prenatal care, 23.9 percent had an intermediate level of care, and 7.9 percent of all pregnant women had inadequate care.*

Trends in the use of prenatal care from 1969 to 1980 show steady improvement in the percentage of births to mothers obtaining prenatal care in the first trimester of pregnancy. Since 1980, however, this percentage has remained stable or decreased. Among black women, declines in early use of prenatal care were registered in 1981, 1982, and 1985.

More troubling is that since 1980, there has been an increase in the percentage of births to women with late or no prenatal care. Although this

---

*In this summary, as in the full report, the terms "adequate, intermediate, and inadequate" prenatal care refer to the classification scheme developed by Kessner, and the terms "early, delayed, and late" refer to prenatal care that begins in the first, second, and third trimesters of pregnancy, respectively. The term "insufficient prenatal care" is a general label used to describe care that is neither adequate nor begun early in pregnancy. All such terminology is discussed in detail in Chapter 1.

trend applies to all races, the increase is more pronounced among black women. In 1981, 8.8 percent of births to black women were in this category; by 1985, 10.3 percent were.

These trends present important challenges to public policy and to the health care system for several reasons. First, there is widespread agreement that prenatal care is an effective intervention, strongly and clearly associated with improved pregnancy outcomes; moreover, available evidence suggests that prenatal care is especially important for women at increased medical or social risk, or both. Second, prenatal care is cost-effective. In a 1985 report, for example, the Institute of Medicine calculated that each dollar spent on providing more adequate prenatal care to low-income, poorly educated women could reduce total expenditures for direct medical care of their low birthweight infants by $3.38 during the first year of life; the savings would result from a reduced rate of low birthweight. Finally, the importance of prenatal care is confirmed by international comparisons. Many other countries (particularly Japan and most Western European countries) provide prenatal care to pregnant women as a form of social investment, with minimal barriers or preconditions in place. As a consequence, very high proportions of women in these countries begin prenatal care early in pregnancy.

STUDY FOCUS

Faced with evidence of prenatal care's value and cost-effectiveness, and with data revealing poor and declining use of this key service, in the summer of 1986 the Institute of Medicine convened an interdisciplinary committee, the Committee to Study Outreach for Prenatal Care, to study ways of drawing more women into prenatal care early in pregnancy and of sustaining their participation until delivery. The Committee was asked to focus particularly on outreach as a means for increasing the use of prenatal services. In keeping with conventional understanding, outreach was defined in the study to include various ways of identifying pregnant women and linking them to prenatal care (casefinding) and services helping them remain in care once enrolled (social support).

The Committee's work, however, and the resulting report were not confined to outreach. It became evident early in the study that this service cannot be studied in isolation from the larger maternity care system within which it occurs and that, as a result, the study had to embrace aspects of the surrounding environment. The Committee's conclusions and recommendations are not limited to outreach, therefore, but also touch on issues of maternity care financing and organization. The report's major sections cover demographic risk factors, barriers to the use of prenatal care, women's perceptions of barriers to care, providers' opinions about the factors that account for delayed care, multivariate analysis of predictors of prenatal care use, and lessons learned from a variety of programs that attempt to improve utilization of this basic health service.

DEMOGRAPHIC RISK FACTORS

Several demographic risk factors are closely associated with insufficient prenatal care:

Minority Status Among white women giving birth in 1985, 79.4 percent began care in the first trimester of pregnancy and 4.7 percent received late or no care. Black women were far less likely than white women to begin care early (61.8 percent) and twice as likely to receive late or no care (10.1 percent versus 4.7 percent). Hispanic mothers are substantially less likely than non-Hispanic white mothers to begin prenatal care early and are three times as likely to obtain late or no care. Moreover, Hispanic mothers as a group are more likely than non-Hispanic black mothers to begin care late or not at all. American Indian women are more likely than either white or black women to obtain late or no care.

Age Young mothers are at high risk of obtaining late or no prenatal care, with the greatest risk for the youngest mothers, those under 15. Mothers age 40 and over are less likely than mothers age 25 to 39 to begin care in the first trimester and more likely to obtain care late or not at all.

Education Timing of the first prenatal visit correlates highly with educational attainment. In 1985, 88 percent of mothers with at least some college education began care early in pregnancy, compared with 58 percent of mothers who had less than a high school education. The probability that a pregnant woman will obtain care late or not at all decreases steadily as her educational level increases.

Birth order The more children a woman has had, the more likely she is to obtain insufficient care or none at all. In 1985, nearly 5 percent of both first and second children were born to mothers who obtained late or no care. About 6 percent of third births fell into this category, however, and the numbers increased to 9 and 14 percent for fourth and fifth children, respectively.

Marital status Unmarried mothers are more than three times as likely as married mothers to obtain late or no prenatal care (13.0 and 3.4 percent, respectively, in 1985). Unmarried white mothers are almost four times as likely as married white mothers to obtain late or no care; and unmarried black mothers are twice as likely as married black mothers to obtain late or no care. Among unmarried mothers, women of Hispanic origin are most likely to obtain late or no care, followed by white non-Hispanic and then black non-Hispanic mothers. The correlation of unmarried status with insufficient prenatal care has become more salient in recent years as childbearing among unmarried women has increased, reaching an all-time high of 828,000 births (about 22 percent of all births) in 1985.

Income   Poverty is one of the most important correlates of insufficient prenatal care. Women below the federal poverty level consistently show higher rates of late or no care and lower rates of early care than women with larger incomes. Given that one-third of all U.S. births are to women with incomes less than 150 percent of the federal poverty level, the consistent correlation of low income with insufficient prenatal care is of major importance and forms the basis of many Committee recommendations.

Geographic location   Insufficient prenatal care is concentrated in certain geographic areas, most often inner cities and isolated rural areas. States vary in their rates of early and late entry into care, and great diversity in use of prenatal care can exist within states, counties, cities and even neighborhoods.

Barriers to the Use of Prenatal Care

Four categories of obstacles to full participation in prenatal care can be described: (1) a set of financial barriers ranging from problems in private insurance and Medicaid to the complete absence of health insurance; (2) inadequate capacity in the prenatal care systems relied on by many low-income women; (3) problems in the organization, practices, and atmosphere of prenatal services themselves; and (4) cultural and personal factors that can limit use of care.

Financial Barriers

Women with *private health insurance* are more likely to obtain adequate prenatal care than uninsured or Medicaid-enrolled women, but many women do not have access to employer-based group coverage (the most common means of obtaining private insurance). Even when such coverage is available, the cost to the employee may be too high to enroll or coverage may not include maternity care or require substantial cost sharing.

The *Medicaid* program is the largest single source of health care financing for the poor and is believed to be primarily responsible for the increased use of medical services by low-income individuals since its enactment in 1965. Natality data from 1969 (shortly after Medicaid was enacted) and 1980 show significant increases in the proportion of pregnant women seeking care in the first trimester. Medicaid has been particularly important in increasing minority access to prenatal care.

Despite such favorable trends, data also show that women covered by Medicaid do not obtain prenatal care as early in pregnancy or make as many visits to providers as women with private insurance. At least three reasons have been offered for this differential. The Medicaid enrollment process is so time-consuming that a woman may be well into her pregnancy before her eligibility is established. Second, Medicaid-insured women rely more heavily on clinics for prenatal care, and these clinics are often overburdened and unable to schedule appointments promptly; similarly, the number of physicians accepting Medicaid-enrolled pregnant women has always been limited and in some areas is decreasing. Finally, women on Medicaid are characterized by numerous demographic factors associated with insufficient prenatal care, including being unmarried, having less education, being under 20, and being in fair or poor health. Given these attributes of the Medicaid population, health insurance alone is unlikely to close the gap between their use of health services and that of more affluent women with private coverage.

A substantial proportion of the poor is not covered by Medicaid. In fact, in 1988, the average income eligibility ceiling for Medicaid was only 49 percent of the federal poverty level. In addition, the proportion of the poor covered by Medicaid has decreased: it is estimated that in 1976, 65 percent of the poor were covered by Medicaid; in 1984, the comparable figure was 38 percent. Congress has expanded Medicaid eligibility for pregnant women through numerous laws passed in the mid-1980s. One of the most important reforms in these laws severs the link between Medicaid and AFDC (that is, Aid to Families with Dependent Children—welfare). Thus, some women may now become eligible for Medicaid even if they are not eligible for AFDC, and states have the opportunity to increase Medicaid eligibility for targeted subgroups, and to receive federal matching funds, without increasing AFDC program costs.

Between the group covered by private insurance and the group enrolled in Medicaid are the *uninsured*. By the mid-1980s, more than 37 million Americans were completely uninsured, and women of childbearing age are disproportionately represented among them. An estimated 26 percent of women of reproductive age (14.6 million) have no insurance to cover maternity care, and two-thirds of these (9.5 million) have no health insurance at all. Of poor women, 35 percent are completely uninsured.

Women with no insurance face significant obstacles to obtaining prenatal services and must rely on free or reduced-cost care from willing private physicians or from health department clinics and other settings usually financed by public funds. Unfortunately, the proportion of women age 15 to 44 who are uninsured is likely to grow.

Inadequate System Capacity

Numerous reports document inadequate numbers of, and long waiting times for appointments at, such facilities as Community Health Centers and health department clinics—settings that have traditionally provided prenatal care to those unable or unwilling to use the private care system. Similarly, there appears to be a growing demand for prenatal services in clinics—a picture consistent with the increasing number of women of reproductive age without adequate private health insurance and the decreasing number of private providers caring for Medicaid-enrolled and other low-income women. Adequate or even excess capacity can exist for affluent women in the same geographic area as inadequate capacity for low-income women.

Limited availability of maternity care providers is a major contributor to the capacity problem. Many areas of the country have few or no obstetricians in practice. Large numbers of obstetricians will not take patients who are uninsured, and many do not accept Medicaid clients. An important reason for this disinclination is that Medicaid reimbursement rates are often very low and represent only a fraction of cost or of privately reimbursed fees. The increase in malpractice insurance premiums and a growing concern about the risk of malpractice litigation are also associated with the increasing number of providers who have discontinued or appreciably reduced their obstetrical practice. In some communities, particularly those with poorer populations and no teaching or public facilities, obstetrical care may be disappearing entirely.

Organization, Practices, and Atmosphere of Prenatal Services

Use of prenatal care can also be limited by the way services are organized and provided at the delivery site. Common barriers include inadequate coordination of services (such as poor links among health department clinics, private physicians, and such other service systems as welfare and housing); problems in securing Medicaid (the application and enrollment process can often be time-consuming and difficult, and eligible women may know little about the program or how and where to apply); and a host of classic access barriers well known to limit use of not only prenatal care but also health services generally (including transportation problems, difficulties in arranging child care, service hours that do not accommodate the schedules of women who work or go to school, long waits in clinics, communication problems between providers and clients, language and cultural barriers, unpleasant surroundings, and lack of easily accessible information about where to go for prenatal care).

Cultural and Personal Barriers

Use of prenatal care can be limited by a woman's attitudes toward her pregnancy and toward prenatal care, her cultural values and beliefs, a variety of other personal characteristics often called life-style, and certain psychological attributes. Attitudes toward pregnancy that may influence efforts to seek prenatal care include whether the pregnancy is planned or unplanned and whether the woman views her pregnancy positively or negatively. These are particularly important issues because more than half of all pregnancies in the United States are unplanned. In addition, not all women believe that prenatal care is important and worth the effort to seek it out. Some believe that care is needed only if a pregnant woman feels ill; among some cultures, pregnancy is regarded as a healthy condition not requiring medical treatment or advice from a health care provider. A few women may actually be unaware of what prenatal care is or what the signs of pregnancy are. Previous, unsatisfying experiences with prenatal services may also act as a deterrent.

Pregnant women may avoid prenatal care because they fear providers or medical procedures, because they fear others' reactions to the pregnancy, or because they fear that their illegal status in the country will be discovered. Pregnant women who are aware that such personal habits as drug and alcohol abuse, heavy smoking, and eating disorders place their health and that of their babies at risk may also avoid care because they anticipate sanction or pressure to change. Unfortunately, numerous reports detail alarming increases in the proportion of women, including pregnant women, who abuse heroin and cocaine and in the number of babies born with varying degrees of addiction.

Having friends and family to offer emotional support and tangible assistance, and having well-developed skills in overcoming isolation, may minimize or eliminate barriers to prenatal care; lack of these assets, particularly when combined with poverty, may constitute a barrier to care in and of itself. Homeless women, for example, have very poor rates of prenatal care use. Stress, depression, and denial may also decrease a woman's ability to seek prenatal care.

BARRIERS TO CARE: WOMEN'S AND PROVIDERS' PERSPECTIVES

Although numerous barriers to prenatal care have been noted in many studies, the relative importance of these barriers to women themselves is not as well documented. Few reports on obstacles to prenatal care cite "consumer" views, and programs aimed at increasing participation in care are often designed without careful assessment of women's experiences with maternity care. To help fill this gap, the Committee synthesized the findings of numerous studies of women who had obtained insufficient prenatal services and who had been queried about factors they felt had caused their delay in entering care.

Financial barriers—particularly inadequate or no insurance and limited personal funds—were the most important obstacles reported in 15 studies of women who received insufficient care. Transportation problems also emerged as major barriers. A very important message from these studies is that many women who obtained insufficient care attach a low value to prenatal services. Other barriers that frequently appeared include some variation on "I didn't know I was pregnant," inhospitable institutional practices (such as inconvenient hours and long waits in clinics), limited provider availability, and dislike or fear of prenatal care.

In six studies of women who obtained no prenatal care at all, financial barriers were again the most commonly cited obstacle. The second most common was a low value placed on prenatal care. Other barriers frequently reported by these women include transportation difficulties, inhospitable institutional practices, and a dislike or fear of prenatal services.

The Committee reviewed three studies that assessed teenagers' views of barriers to prenatal care. These studies suggest that such internal factors as fear, shame, and denial may well overshadow financial obstacles to care, at least at the outset. Given their youth, adolescents may also be particularly likely to know little about prenatal care and to place a low value on what they do know of it. Common sense suggests that when adolescents actually try to seek care, the problems of limited personal funds and no insurance also loom large.

A 1987 survey conducted by the American College of Obstetricians and Gynecologists studied whether obstetricians see barriers to prenatal care in roughly the same way their clients do. In general, the survey found notable agreement between clients and providers. The most important obstacle to care cited by the obstetricians was financial problems followed by a belief that prenatal care is not necessary.

MULTIVARIATE ANALYSIS

The Committee reviewed 12 studies that used multivariate analysis to determine predictors of prenatal care use. The value of this analytic technique is that it can consider the combined effects of demographic risk factors, general barriers to care, and the reasons offered by women about why they obtained insufficient care. Although results of the 12 analyses could not be pooled, several themes emerged. Poverty (especially as represented by inadequate or no health insurance) was a consistently important predictor of insufficient care. Except for race, all of the other demographic risk factors noted earlier were also found to predict insufficient care in many of the studies, along with unintended pregnancy and a low opinion of prenatal services. Despite the clear value of these studies in defining key risk factors and in defining target groups, there is need for more sophisticated understanding of the factors influencing use of this key health service.

IMPROVING THE USE OF PRENATAL CARE: PROGRAM EXPERIENCE

The Committee studied 31 programs that have tried to improve participation in prenatal care. These programs were divided into five groups, depending on their major emphasis:

1. reducing financial obstacles to care;
2. increasing the basic capacity of the prenatal care system relied on by many low-income women;
3. improving institutional practices to make services more easily accessible and acceptable to clients;
4. identifying women in need of prenatal care (casefinding) through a wide variety of methods, including hotlines, community canvassing using outreach workers or other paraprofessional personnel, cross-agency referrals, and the provision of incentives; and
5. providing social support to encourage continuation in prenatal care and smooth the transition into parenthood.

The last two categories include the majority of activities generally viewed as outreach. Consonant with the Committee's charge, a special effort was made to examine programs in these categories.

The objective of studying a given program was not merely to understand its approach to improving access, but also to determine which activities appeared effective, with what populations, and under what circumstances. Program effectiveness was measured in terms of the month of pregnancy in which prenatal care was begun or the number of prenatal visits or both. Programs that had assessed their impact using only birth outcome measures (such as length of gestation, birthweight, Apgar score, or infant mortality) were excluded from the group of programs studied.

Unfortunately, the data available to judge program effectiveness are rarely excellent and often inadequate. Most programs have few funds for evaluation; when unrestricted dollars are available, service demands usually take precedence. Even the few evaluated programs reviewed by the Committee seldom used randomization techniques or other strong research designs to assess program effects. Selection bias, in particular, clouds most evaluations. Moreover, because many programs are complex, it is often difficult to distinguish the impact of individual elements.

This is not to say, however, that no judgment could be made regarding program effectiveness. The Committee concluded that each of the five types of programs can succeed in bringing women into prenatal care and maintaining their participation. It is nonetheless true that the success of many programs is modest, often because they are anomalies in a complicated, fragmented network of maternity services characterized by pervasive financial and institutional obstacles to care. The Committee was struck by the amount of effort these disparate programs involve, the degree of personal dedication required of their leaders, and the difficulties many have had to overcome to make progress. The goal of early and continuous use of prenatal care by pregnant women may seem straightforward and obviously sensible, but attaining it in the United States at present is proving to be an arduous task.

More specific conclusions were also drawn about the five types of programs. With regard to the first category—removing financial barriers to care—the Committee noted how few programs could be identified that take this direct approach to improving participation in prenatal care, despite the salience of financial obstacles. Most try to ease financial barriers by enlarging the clinic systems relied on by low-income pregnant women, rather than by enabling them to use provider systems already in place, including physicians in private practice.

The program data also suggest that increasing the capacity of the prenatal care systems relied on by low-income women can improve utilization among this population. Nurse–practitioners, certified nurse–midwives, and other mid-level practitioners are often central to this approach.

With regard to the third programmatic approach—revising internal procedures and policies—the Committee found very persuasive data that institutional modification can improve participation in prenatal care substantially. The programs reviewed in this category underscore the importance of how clients are treated, what the clinic or office procedures are, and what the atmosphere of the setting is.

The fourth cluster of programs reveals great variety in casefinding methods. Data from projects that conduct casefinding with outreach workers and similar personnel suggest that the number of clients recruited is often low and that the cost per client enrolled can be very high, particularly in highly mobile urban settings; nonetheless, outreach workers can sometimes find the hardest-to-reach women. Program managers report that outreach workers can be difficult to recruit, train, supervise, and motivate, and that only the most skilled and persistent are likely to succeed. Both funders and program planners tend to underestimate the costs and complexity of using this means of casefinding.

Hotlines appear to be meeting a real need and their success shows that the telephone has great potential for casefinding. When hotline workers follow up on referrals and attempt to solve the problems faced by their callers in securing care, they can help to overcome major barriers. Casefinding through cross-program referrals can also improve participation in prenatal care. Close cooperation between prenatal services and pregnancy testing services, pediatric services, and WIC sites (that is, sites administering the Special Supplemental Food Program for Women, Infants, and Children) seems particularly useful.

The Committee found little evidence that incentives in kind or in cash brought women into care, although the amount of data available in this area is extremely limited. Programs that use this approach generally report that the women are appreciative, but program staff do not think the incentives themselves are the primary factor in initiating or maintaining care.

The final category of projects reviewed emphasizes social support, principally as a means of encouraging women to continue care. Program data indicate that this approach can result in an increased number of prenatal visits. Populations at greatest risk of insufficient prenatal care, such as young teenagers and low-income minority women, often require significant social and emotional support, information, advice, and caring. Those providing such assistance through health care or social service agencies are well positioned to urge pregnant clients to seek and remain in prenatal care and to comply with the recommendations of their health care providers.

Program Implementation and Evaluation

Many program leaders face major difficulties in implementing and maintaining programs. Problems fall into five groups: planning programs, finding financial and community support, dealing with bureaucracies, recruiting and keeping personnel, and sustaining momentum. The Committee also found that virtually all programs struggle with evaluation— what to evaluate, how to build data collection into routine program activities, how to enlist staff in the process of evaluation when providing service is their primary focus, and, above all, how to find adequate money, staff, and time to do high-quality evaluation studies. Some programs that believed they were evaluating their activities properly were found, on closer examination, to be using inadequate evaluation designs, yielding data of limited value. The net result is that the quality of most program evaluation reviewed by the Committee was poor and that considerable energy was being wasted.

CONCLUSIONS AND RECOMMENDATIONS

The data and program experience reviewed by the Committee reveal a maternity care system* that is fundamentally flawed, fragmented, and overly complex. Unlike many European nations, the United States has no direct, straightforward system for making maternity services easily accessible. Although well-insured, affluent women can be reasonably certain of receiving appropriate health care during pregnancy and childbirth, many women cannot share this expectation. Low-income women, women who are uninsured or underinsured, teenagers, inner-city and rural residents, certain minority groups, and other high-risk populations are likely to experience significant problems in obtaining necessary maternity services.

The Committee concludes that in the long run, the best prospects for improving use of prenatal care—and reversing current declines—lie in reorganizing the nation's maternity care system. Although a new system may include some elements of the existing one, the Committee specifically recommends against the current practice of making incremental changes in programs already in place. Instead, it argues for fundamental reform. Several ways are available for designing the specific components of a new system, but no such work should proceed until the nation's leaders first make a commitment to enact substantial changes. A deeper commitment to family planning services and education should accompany improvements in the maternity care system.

In the short term, the Committee urges strengthening existing systems through which women secure prenatal services. This includes simultaneous actions to:

1. remove financial barriers to care;
2. make certain that basic system capacity is adequate for all women;
3. improve the policies and practices that shape prenatal services at the delivery site; and
4. increase public information and education about prenatal care.

Federal leadership of this four-part program is essential, supplemented by state action to ensure the availability of prenatal services to all residents.

---

*That is, the complicated network of publicly and privately financed services through which women obtain prenatal, labor and delivery, and postpartum care.

Even if all four system changes were implemented, however, there would still be some women without sufficient care because of extreme social isolation, youth, fear or denial, drug addiction, cultural factors, or other reasons. For these women, there is a clear need for casefinding and social support to locate and enroll them in prenatal services and to encourage continuation in care once begun. These outreach services, supplementing a well-designed, highly accessible system of prenatal services, can help draw the most hard-to-reach women into care.

Unfortunately, though, outreach is often undertaken without first making certain that the basic maternity care system is accessible and responsive to women's needs. Too often, communities organize outreach to help women over and around major obstacles to care rather than removing the obstacles themselves. To fund outreach in isolation and hope that it alone will accomplish major improvements in the use of prenatal services is naive and wasteful.

In support of this general view, the Committee makes a number of recommendations regarding program management, evaluation, and research. The Committee concludes that not all programs should have to muster the funds and expertise to conduct formal evaluation studies. For those that choose to do so, a higher quality of effort is needed than that exhibited by most of the programs reviewed. With regard to research, the Committee specifically urges that no more research be conducted to demonstrate the importance of financial and other institutional barriers to care. The Committee does, however, suggest six specific research topics (see recommendation 14 below) and recommends that the current practice of securing funds for services under the guise of research cease.

SPECIFIC RECOMMENDATIONS

The full report includes 14 major recommendations; most have one or more subsidiary recommendations not included in this brief summary.

1. We recommend that the nation adopt as a new social norm the principle that all pregnant women—not only the affluent—should be provided access to prenatal, labor and delivery, and postpartum services appropriate to their need. Actions in all sectors of society, and clear leadership from the public sector especially, will be required for this principle to become a clear, explicit, and widely shared value.

2. We recommend that the President, members of Congress, and other national leaders in both the public and private sectors commit themselves openly and unequivocally to designing a new maternity care system—or systems—dedicated to drawing all women into prenatal care and providing them with an appropriate array of health and social services throughout

pregnancy, childbirth, and the postpartum period. Although a new system might build on existing arrangements, long-term solutions require fundamental reforms, not incremental changes in existing programs.

3. We recommend that more immediate efforts to increase participation in prenatal care emphasize four goals: eliminating financial barriers to care, making certain that the capacity of the maternity care system is adequate, improving the policies and practices that shape prenatal services at the site where they are provided, and increasing public information about prenatal care. (In recommendations 5 through 8, each of these four goals is developed more fully.)

4. We recommend that the federal government provide increased leadership, financial support, and incentives to help states and communities meet the four goals we advocate (recommendation 3). In a parallel effort, states should accept responsibility for ensuring that prenatal care is genuinely available to all pregnant women in the state, relying on federal assistance as needed in meeting this responsibility.

5. We recommend that top priority be given to eliminating financial barriers to prenatal care. (More specific recommendations are directed toward Medicaid, the various federal grant programs, state and local health departments, and private insurance.)

6. We recommend that public and private leaders designing policies to draw pregnant women into prenatal care make certain that services are plentiful enough in a community to enable all women to secure appointments within two weeks with providers close to their homes. (Numerous methods for achieving this goal are suggested.)

7. We recommend that those responsible for providing prenatal services periodically review and revise office or clinic procedures to make certain that access is easy and prompt, bureaucratic requirements minimal, and the atmosphere welcoming. Equally important, services should be provided to encourage women to continue care. Follow-up of missed appointments should be routine, and additional social supports should be available where needed. (Many suggestions are made to improve institutional practices at the delivery site.)

8. We recommend that public and private groups—government, foundations, health services agencies, professional societies, and others—invest in a long-term, high-quality public information campaign to educate Americans about the importance of prenatal care for healthy mothers and infants and the need to begin such care early in pregnancy. The campaign should carry its message to schools, the media, family planning and other health care settings, social service networks, and places of employment. Additional campaigns should be aimed at the groups at highest risk for insufficient care. Whether directed at the entire population or a specific subgroup, public information campaigns should always include specific

instructions on where to go or whom to call to arrange for prenatal services.

9. We recommend that initiatives to increase use of prenatal care not rely on casefinding and social support to correct the major financial and institutional barriers that currently impede access. Rather, outreach should be only one component of a well-designed, well-functioning system and should be targeted toward women who remain unserved despite easily accessible services. Outreach should only be funded when it is linked to a highly accessible system of prenatal services, or, at a minimum, when it is part of a comprehensive plan to strengthen the system, emphasizing the four areas previously described.

10. We recommend that in communities where financial and institutional barriers have been removed, or as part of a comprehensive plan to do so, at least five kinds of casefinding be considered for their compatibility with a program's goals and constraints: (a) telephone hotline and referral services that can make prenatal appointments during the initial call and can provide assistance to callers in arranging needed maternity, health, and social services; (b) television and, in particular, radio spots to announce specific services, coordinated with posters displayed in the mass transit system; (c) efforts to encourage current program participants to recruit additional participants from their friends, neighbors, and relatives; (d) strong referral ties between prenatal programs and a variety of other systems in which pregnant women at risk for insufficient care may be found: family planning clinics, schools, housing programs, WIC agencies, welfare and unemployment offices, churches and community service groups, shelters for the homeless, the police and corrections systems, substance-abuse programs and treatment centers, and other health and social service networks; and (e) outreach workers who canvass in carefully defined target areas and seek clients among well-defined target populations. Whatever the method used, casefinding should be directed toward high-risk groups and areas. This requires that program leaders pinpoint the sociodemographic characteristics and geographic locations of women who obtain insufficient prenatal care.

11. We recommend that programs providing prenatal services to high-risk, often low-income groups include social support services to help maintain participation in care and arrange for additional services as needed. Home visiting is an important form of social support and should be available in programs caring for high-risk women.

12. We recommend that programs to improve participation in prenatal care invest generously in planning and needs assessment. Doing so will require a deeper appreciation, among funders in particular, of the time needed for responsible, intelligent program design and planning. Substantial improvements in the use of prenatal care (or in other measures of

outcome such as low birthweight or infant mortality) should not be expected too soon.

13. We recommend that early in a program's course its directors decide whether it is to be primarily a service program (with data collected mainly to help in program development and monitoring) or whether it is also to test an idea in the field. The latter type requires ample funding if the evaluation is to be sound; it also requires experts in program evaluation and sophisticated systems for data collection—resources that must be built into the program from the outset.

14. We recommend that *in communities where financial and institutional obstacles to care have been significantly lowered*, research be undertaken on several topics: (a) Why do some pregnant women register late—or not at all—for prenatal care, even when financial and institutional barriers are ostensibly absent? In particular, what are the emotional and attitudinal factors that limit participation in care? (b) How can the content of prenatal care be revised to encourage women to seek such care early in pregnancy? (c) What casefinding techniques are most helpful in identifying very high-risk groups (such as low-income multiparous teenagers) and linking them to prenatal services? (d) What are the costs associated with various forms of casefinding and social support? (e) What are the most effective ways to forge links between physicians in private practice and community agencies providing the ancillary health and social services that high-risk women often need? and (f) How is access to maternity services being affected by such recent developments as the decreased ability of hospitals to finance care for indigent patients through cost shifting, the increase in corporate ownership of hospitals, the gradual expansion of the DRG (diagnosis-related groups) system beyond the Medicare program, and the increasing profit orientation of the health care sector generally?

Introduction

In 1985, approximately one-fourth of all infants in the United States were born to women who did not begin prenatal care in the first 3 months (or trimester) of pregnancy; a larger proportion—almost one-third—were born to women who did not obtain the amount of care currently recommended by the American College of Obstetricians and Gynecologists.[1] More than 5 percent were born to women who began care only in the third trimester of pregnancy or had no care at all. For certain groups, these percentages were even higher. For example, only 47 percent of black teenagers began care in the first trimester of pregnancy, and 14 percent obtained either no care or care only in the third trimester.[2]

Unfortunately, the steady increase during the 1970s in the proportion of women who begin prenatal care in the first trimester of pregnancy has ceased in the 1980s. And in 1985, for the sixth consecutive year, no progress was made in reducing the percentage of infants born to women who begin care only in the third trimester or not at all. For blacks, the size of this group actually appears to be increasing. In 1980, 8.8 percent of black infants were born to mothers who had third trimester or no prenatal care; by 1985, this number had grown to 10.3 percent.[3]

These disturbing trends present important challenges to public policy and to the health care system for several reasons. First, there is widespread agreement that prenatal care is an effective intervention, strongly and clearly associated with improved pregnancy outcomes. Because randomized clinical trials are precluded on ethical grounds, incontrovertible scientific proof of this effectiveness is not available; nevertheless, exhaustive reviews of the literature and recent analyses continue to document the value of this basic health service.[4,5] Declines in rates of maternal mortality, infant mortality, and low birthweight have been repeatedly associated with full participation in comprehensive prenatal care that is well connected to hospital-based services for labor and delivery and for neonatal care. Available evidence suggests that prenatal care is especially important for women at increased medical or social risk, or both.

The importance of prenatal care also derives from its cost-effectiveness, particularly for low-income women. For example, in 1985, the Institute of Medicine calculated that each dollar spent on providing more adequate prenatal care to a cohort of low-income, poorly educated women could reduce total expenditures for direct medical care of their low birthweight infants by $3.38 during the first year of life.[6] (The savings would result from a reduced rate of low birthweight.) Other investigators have computed different ratios, but virtually all find evidence of cost-effectiveness.[7–10]

Finally, the importance of prenatal care is confirmed by international comparisons. As discussed by C. Arden Miller in the paper he contributed to this volume and by others,[11] many countries (particularly Japan and most Western European countries) provide prenatal care to pregnant women as a form of social investment. These countries, many of them with fewer resources than the United States, have developed relatively simple, well-functioning maternity systems. Prenatal care, like health services generally, is made readily available with minimal barriers or preconditions in place, and it is closely connected to numerous social and financial supports for pregnant women and young families. Such services are seen as part of a broad social strategy to protect and support childbearing and to produce healthy future generations. As a result of this comprehensive approach, many European countries report that very high proportions of their pregnant women begin prenatal care early in pregnancy; they also report lower rates of infant mortality and low birthweight.[12] While the U.S. Surgeon General has set a goal of reducing the proportion of women who obtain no prenatal care during the first 3 months of pregnancy to 10 percent by 1990, the U.S. Department of Health and Human Services recently acknowledged that, "based on progress to date, it appears unlikely that this objective will be met."[13]

This country's limited progress in extending prenatal care is only part of a larger problem of poor access to health services for low-income and minority populations. In the face of an increasingly competitive, profit-oriented medical care system, the United States has failed to find adequate ways to finance health care for the poor. In 1988, socioeconomic status remains a major determinant of both health status and use of medical services. Moreover, there is some evidence that access to health care may

be deteriorating for poor, minority, and uninsured Americans.[14,15] Igelhart
has stated:

The goal of providing quality medical care to the entire population of a vast country
that prizes limited government, freedom, and individualism has remained elusive.
Substantial resources have been committed to the task, and many citizens are prepared
to allocate more, but the results thus far have been less than socially satisfying. To
many millions of Americans, access to medical care remains uncertain or unobtainable,
even though the United States spends more per capita for care than any other
industrialized nation.[16]

STUDY FOCUS

Faced with evidence of prenatal care's value and cost-effectiveness, and
with data revealing poor and declining use of this key service, in the
summer of 1986 the Institute of Medicine convened an interdisciplinary
committee, the Committee to Study Outreach for Prenatal Care, to study
ways of drawing more women into prenatal care early in pregnancy and of
sustaining their participation until delivery. The Committee was asked to
develop recommendations for improving participation in prenatal care,
particularly through "outreach." In keeping with conventional understanding, outreach was defined to include various ways of identifying pregnant
women and linking them to prenatal care (casefinding) and services that
offer support and assistance to help women remain in care once enrolled
(social support).

The special emphasis on outreach grew out of several considerations.
First, an earlier Institute of Medicine committee had recommended that
the nature and role of outreach in increasing access to prenatal care be
studied. Concluding that the field was ill-defined, little-understood, and
undervalued, the Committee urged that efforts be made to "assemble and
integrate existing information about outreach approaches and to identify
additional research needs."[17]

Second, many community-based prenatal care programs rely heavily on
outreach to improve access, believing that it is effective in bringing women
into care and maintaining their participation. Despite its potential importance, however, outreach is often discontinued—"cut first"—when health
services face fiscal difficulties. The vulnerability of outreach is not
surprising, given the unwillingness of most insurance systems to cover its
costs, the scant and widely scattered data on its effectiveness, its relatively
low status as a health service, and the low pay and training often provided
to its practitioners.

Finally, the Committee was asked to concentrate especially on outreach
because it has attracted so little scholarship. It was hoped that assembling

a wide variety of materials on prenatal outreach would increase the interest of health services researchers (and those who fund their work) in studying this neglected field.

The Committee's work and this volume, however, were not confined to outreach for prenatal care. The Committee realized early in the study that this service cannot not be studied in isolation from the larger maternity care system* within which it occurs and that, as a consequence, the study's boundaries had to expand beyond outreach. At least four factors led to this broadened scope of study. First, many projects labelled as outreach are deeply involved in such problem-solving activities as helping women arrange financing for hospital-based childbirth—activities that are not included in conventional understandings of outreach. Second, the goals and content of outreach programs are so heavily influenced by the larger systems within which they operate that it would have been difficult, if not useless, to analyze them separately. Third, outreach is not the only way to accomplish the goals of earlier registration and improved continuation in prenatal care; other approaches can have the same effect and thus merit study. (These other methods include reducing financial barriers to care, making certain that system capacity is adequate, and improving the policies and practices that shape prenatal services at the delivery site.) Fourth and finally, the larger maternity care system was considered because it makes little sense to study ways of drawing women into care if the system they enter cannot, or will not, be responsive to their needs.

In this context, one issue deserves particular attention. Although the gap between prenatal services and hospitalization for labor and delivery might be considered well outside the jurisdiction of this Committee, it is too important to ignore in any policy analysis of maternity services. Every pregnant woman needs not only prenatal care, but also a safe, well-equipped setting in which to deliver her infant. Despite the clear need for such a continuum of care, there is ample evidence that the ties between prenatal and delivery services are often tenuous.[18] In some areas of the country, for example, women may receive prenatal care at Community Health Centers or health department clinics but deliver in hospitals without their prenatal records available, simply because of inadequate systems for transferring records among providers.[19] Moreover, obtaining prenatal services does not lead automatically to admission at a hospital of choice for labor and delivery, because many institutions require large preadmission deposits or create other barriers to admission. (For example, in Brownsville, Texas, about 40 percent of women deliver out of hospital—

---

*That is, the complicated network of publicly and privately financed services through which women obtain prenatal, labor and delivery, and postpartum care.

compared with a 1 percent rate nationally—because the area's two for-profit hospitals require large preadmission deposits and have been reluctant to contract with the state for obstetrical care for low-income women.[20]) Similarly, state programs that fund prenatal services often do not include funding for labor and delivery. A 1986 survey of 51 state maternal and child health agencies found that few state agencies have resources to help uninsured and other poor women pay for hospitalization for delivery. Only 23 states reported that they had funding for inpatient obstetrical care; 16 reported that existing funds were restricted to women who participated in designated maternity programs or were identified as high-risk prior to delivery. No state reported a program to fund hospital services for all uninsured pregnant women.[21]

These major flaws and gaps in the organization of maternity services provided additional impetus for the Committee's decision to enlarge its scope of study beyond the issue of outreach. One consequence of the expanded boundaries is that the Committee's conclusions and recommendations (Chapter 5) are not limited to outreach, but also touch on issues of maternity care financing and organization.

It is important to add that even with this larger scope of study, the report focuses on a limited topic. In particular, by concentrating on maternity care, other women's health services are largely overlooked, as are important issues of women's health status. For example, the poor coordination that often exists among family planning services, sexually transmitted disease services, general medical care and maternity services is addressed only briefly in this report. Although such limits are appropriate given the Committee's mandate, it is important to acknowledge them. Women need good health care whether pregnant or not, and plans to improve maternity services should always be developed within this broader context.

STUDY METHOD

The Committee surveyed existing or recently completed prenatal care programs in order to understand the range of approaches currently being used to increase participation in care, and to determine if data were available to judge their effect. The programs were divided by the Committee into five broad categories, and one or more programs in each category was reviewed:

1. reducing the financial obstacles to care encountered by poor and uninsured women through provision of insurance or other sources of payment;

2. increasing the capacity of the prenatal care system relied on by many low-income women, which includes health department clinics, the network of

private physicians who care for Medicaid-enrolled and other low-income women, hospital outpatient clinics, Community Health Centers, and similar settings;

3. improving institutional practices to make services more easily accessible and acceptable to clients;

4. conducting active casefinding through such methods as hotlines, community canvassing via outreach workers or other paraprofessional personnel, cross-agency referrals, and the provision of incentives;

5. providing social support to encourage continuation in prenatal care and, more generally, to increase the probability of healthy pregnancies and smooth the transition into parenthood.

The last two categories include the majority of activities generally considered outreach. In keeping with its charge, the Committee made a special effort to examine programs in those categories.

The objective of studying a given program was not merely to understand its approach to improving access, but also to determine which activities appeared effective, with what populations, and under what circumstances. The Committee posed the question: What is the evidence that the approach leads to earlier registration in prenatal care, to participation in care by women previously unserved, to improved continuation in care once begun, or any combination of these? The Committee also examined the environment in which programs had developed, the problems they faced, and the constraints on further expansion.

An important part of the Committee's review of program data was a workshop held in May 1987 in which members talked in depth with the leaders of eight programs that use various means to improve participation in prenatal care. This opportunity to discuss in detail a number of issues that had emerged from written reports provided valuable insight into the history and current forces shaping such programs.

In addition to reviewing project data, the Committee considered a variety of other information sources. It conducted a literature review, arranged for numerous commissioned and contributed papers, and had many informal conversations and correspondence with prenatal care providers, policymakers, and researchers.

ORGANIZATION OF THE REPORT

This volume begins with a brief summary that covers not only the body of the report, but also key themes in their introduction. Chapter 1 presents a demographic analysis of who does and does not obtain prenatal care and contains trends in utilization. Chapter 2 summarizes the literature on barriers to prenatal services. Chapter 3 synthesizes 17 studies of women's views about obstacles to care and discusses 12 recent multivariate analyses of predictors of prenatal care use. Chapter 4 presents lessons learned from the Committee's review of 31 programs that attempt to draw women into care early in pregnancy and sustain their participation. Chapter 5 presents the Committee's conclusions and recommendations; these are directed toward those involved in national, state, and local health policy; those who provide maternity services; health services researchers; and leaders in the private sector, particularly those in foundations who fund maternity care programs and related research. Appendix A describes individually the 31 programs studied. Finally, two commissioned papers are included (Appendixes B and C). One, by Sara Rosenbaum and Dana Hughes of the Children's Defense Fund, delves into the causes and effects of the medical malpractice crisis on poor women's access to care. The other, by C. Arden Miller of the University of North Carolina, contrasts the maternity services available in 10 European countries with those in the United States.

The Value of Prenatal Care: An Underlying Assumption

A very important assumption underlying the entire volume is that prenatal care is a useful and cost-effective service. No effort was made by the Committee to document its benefits further or to defend its value. Nonetheless, the Committee acknowledges that there are many unanswered questions about what the specific components of prenatal services should be and that by focusing primarily on how to draw women into care, the report does not address the important issues of prenatal care's content and quality. The fact that most studies of prenatal services rely on quantitative measures of care, such as number of visits, rather than qualitative ones, increases the tendency in the maternal and child health field generally to overlook these other dimensions. Although the Committee's charge dictated the narrower focus, it is important to state clearly that the quality and content of prenatal services play a large role in their effectiveness, perhaps even more so than the number of visits or the month in which care was begun.

In this context, it is useful to recognize that the term "prenatal care" describes an inexact constellation of procedures and interactions. To some people, the term suggests a minimum set of medical services offered by health care providers on a well-defined schedule, while to others it means those services plus an array of educational, social, and nutritional services provided in a culturally appropriate, flexible fashion. The absence of a clear, universal definition of what constitutes prenatal care is almost certainly at the root of much of the controversy about the content, costs, and effectiveness of this service. Many groups, including the Institute of Medicine, have called for additional research to specify the content of prenatal care as currently offered and to assess the value of each of its components for different groups of women. A final resolution of the question of what is useful in prenatal care, whether defined narrowly or broadly, must await further understanding of the physiology of pregnancy, of threats to maternal and fetal health during pregnancy, and of the specific prenatal interventions needed to minimize these threats.

Progress in this direction is promised by the work of the Public Health Service's Expert Panel on the Content of Prenatal Care. Among other activities, that Panel has proposed a list of outcome variables by which the effectiveness of various aspects of prenatal care could be judged. The list is particularly valuable for its breadth. It suggests that the worth of prenatal care should not be determined solely on the basis of its effect on infant mortality or birthweight—outcomes that have dominated recent discussions of prenatal care—but should consider instead a much broader array of measures. The Panel has proposed that the impact of prenatal care be assessed in terms of maternal, infant, and family health, including, for example, maternal and fetal mortality, the developmental progress of preterm infants, family functioning, planning for future pregnancies, child abuse and neglect, and maternal stress.[22]

While awaiting the Panel's report and further consideration of the content of prenatal care, the Committee has elected to use a broad definition of prenatal care in this volume. Thus it has defined prenatal care to include the diagnosis of pregnancy; the medical, educational, social, and nutritional services needed to enhance the health and well-being of the woman and fetus during pregnancy; and the counseling and assistance required to plan for labor and delivery, postpartum care for the mother, and pediatric care for the newborn.

REFERENCES AND NOTES

1. American College of Obstetricians and Gynecologists. Standards for Obstetric-Gynecologic Services, 6th ed. Washington, D.C., 1985.
2. National Center for Health Statistics. Advance report of final natality statistics, 1985. Monthly Vital Statistics Report, Vol. 36, No. 4 Suppl. DHHS Pub. No. (PHS)87-1120. Hyattsville, Md., 1987.
3. Ibid.
4. Committee to Study the Prevention of Low Birthweight. Preventing Low Birthweight. Washington, D.C.: National Academy Press, 1985.
5. U.S. Congress, Office of Technology Assessment. Healthy Children: Investing in the Future. OTA-H-345. Washington, D.C.: Government Printing Office, 1988.
6. Committee to Study the Prevention of Low Birthweight. Op. cit., pp. 212–237.
7. Moore TR, Origel W, Key TC, and Resnik R. The perinatal and economic impact of prenatal care in a low-socioeconomic population. Am. J. Obstet. Gynecol. 154:29–33, 1986.

8. Corman H and Grossman M. Determinants of neonatal mortality rates in the U.S.—A reduced form model. J. Health Econ. 4:213–236, 1985.
9. Joyce TJ, Corman H, and Grossman M. A cost-effectiveness analysis of strategies to reduce infant mortality. Paper presented at the National Conference on Prenatal Care: New Directions for Federal Policy, sponsored by the Bush Foundation. Washington, D.C., 1986.
10. U.S. Congress, Office of Technology Assessment. *Op. cit.*
11. International Hearings on Infant Mortality, held by the National Commission to Prevent Infant Mortality, United Nations, New York City, 1988.
12. Miller CA. Maternal Health and Infant Survival. Washington, D.C.: National Center for Clinical Infant Programs, 1987.
13. Office of Disease Prevention and Health Promotion. The 1990 Health Objectives for the Nation: A Midcourse Review. Washington, D.C.: U.S. Public Health Service, 1986, p. 51.
14. Freeman HE, Blendon RJ, Aiken LH, Sudman S, Mullinix C, and Corey CR. Americans report on their access to health care. Health Affairs 6(Spring):6–18, 1987, p. 17.
15. Mundinger MO. Health service funding cuts and the declining health of the poor. N. Engl. J. Med. 313:44–47, 1985.
16. Igelhart J.: From the editor. Health Affairs 6(Spring):4–5, 1987, p. 4.
17. Committee to Study the Prevention of Low Birthweight. *Op. cit.*, p. 167.
18. Klerman LV. The maternity care delivery system. Paper presented at the National Conference on Prenatal Care: New Directions for Federal Policy, sponsored by the Bush Foundation. Washington, D.C., 1986.
19. Mayor's Advisory Board on Maternal and Infant Health, District of Columbia. Personal communication, 1988.
20. David Smith, U.S. Public Health Service. Personal communication, 1987.
21. Rosenbaum S, Hughes DC, and Johnson K. Maternal and child health services for medically indigent children and pregnant women. Med. Care 26:315–332, 1988.
22. A final report of the Expert Panel on the Content of Prenatal Care is expected early in 1989.

Chapter

1

———

Who Obtains Insufficient Prenatal Care?

Depending on the measure used, between one-fourth and one-third of all pregnant women in the United States do not obtain early, continuous prenatal care. Women in certain sociodemographic groups and in certain geographic areas are significantly less likely than others to secure care, and in recent years, use of prenatal care has actually declined among some groups. Relying primarily on national vital statistics, this chapter presents data on these correlates and trends, focusing in particular on women who receive little or no care, because such minimal care is strongly associated with poor pregnancy outcomes. It begins with a brief discussion of terminology and methods of measuring prenatal care and then describes current patterns of use, analyzes the relationships among demographic risk factors, and presents trends in the use of prenatal care since 1969.

TERMINOLOGY AND MEASURES

No single specification of the content of prenatal care is unanimously accepted by public health authorities, health care providers, or researchers. The American College of Obstetricians and Gynecologists (ACOG) and a joint working group of representatives from ACOG and from the American Academy of Pediatrics have discussed the goals and content of prenatal care in some detail,[1,2] however, and the Expert Panel on the Content of Prenatal Care and the Preventive Services Task Force (both housed within the U.S. Department of Health and Human Services) promise additional guidance in the future. In the absence of an agreement on the content of prenatal care and because many of its components are difficult to measure, most research on the effectiveness of prenatal services focuses on quantity of care received (such as number of prenatal visits).

Prenatal care differs from other types of health care in the measures used to understand its impact on health outcomes. Most studies of the effectiveness of medical care examine provider actions—for example, did the physician take an adequate history, order the appropriate tests, and conduct the right procedures? By contrast, studies of the role of prenatal care in pregnancy outcome usually examine consumer actions—for example, did the pregnant woman initiate care early, and how many visits did she make? It is unclear why in the field of prenatal services the emphasis is on consumer rather than provider behavior. Exceptions to this method of measuring prenatal care include the work of Morehead, Donaldson, and Seravalli in 1971[3] and, more recently, Hughey in 1986.[4] It is also important to note that various efforts to lower maternal mortality in past years have focused on provider behavior during the prenatal period.

Three measures of the quantity of prenatal care are widely used: (1) the number of visits made throughout pregnancy (frequency), (2) the trimester or month in which care began (timing), and (3) an index relating the frequency and timing of visits to gestational age. This last measure is the basis of the widely used Kessner index,[5] in which a woman's prenatal care is classified as "adequate" if it begins in the first trimester and includes nine or more visits for a pregnancy of 36 or more weeks; "intermediate" if it begins in the second trimester or includes five to eight visits for a pregnancy of 36 or more weeks; or "inadequate" if it begins in the third trimester or includes four or fewer visits for a pregnancy of 34 or more weeks.

All three of these measures tacitly acknowledge the schedule of prenatal visits recommended by ACOG: care beginning as early in the first trimester of pregnancy as possible, with additional visits every 4 weeks for the first 28 weeks of pregnancy, every 2 to 3 weeks for the next 8 weeks, and weekly thereafter until delivery. Such a schedule yields about 12 visits for a 39-week pregnancy, 13 for a 40-week pregnancy, and 14 for a 41-week pregnancy.

All three measures have two major limitations. First, none includes a precise definition of a prenatal visit. A visit for a pregnancy test only, for example, should not be equated with a prenatal care visit, but anecdotal reports suggest that these two distinct events can be confused by women themselves and commingled in data on use of prenatal care. Second, the measures depend either on a woman's recollection of her prenatal visits or on data contained in her medical record. Both sources can be flawed. For example, if a woman changes her source of care during pregnancy, only the date when she started care at the site used immediately before delivery may be noted in her medical records. If these same records are used to complete the birth certificate—the source of data on which most research in this area is based—earlier prenatal visits will be ignored.

The questionable accuracy of birth certificates is substantiated by a study of the 1972 National Natality Survey, in which the number of prenatal visits listed on birth certificates was compared with survey data. Perfect agreement was found in only 16 percent of the cases.[6] In another study, Land and Vaughan reviewed Missouri birth certificate data for 1980 and found that hospitals that obtained information on prenatal care exclusively from the mother reported earlier prenatal care and more visits than those using the prenatal record only or a combination of the prenatal record and information from the mother.[7] Another limitation of birth certificate data is that not all states request information about ethnic origin or the mother's marital status.* Despite such problems, birth certificates remain the best generally available source of data on participation in prenatal care. In particular, they can be used to compare patterns of use across states and populations, and they facilitate analysis of trends.

Each of the three measures also has unique limitations. Counting the number of prenatal visits, while appealing in its simplicity, ignores the distribution of those visits over the pregnancy. The recommended ACOG schedule speaks as much to the timing of prenatal visits as to their absolute number. In particular, counting visits obscures the relationship between prenatal care and preterm delivery. Even if they follow the recommended prenatal schedule, women who deliver prematurely will obviously have fewer prenatal visits than women who deliver at full term. Unless a statistical adjustment is made for length of gestation, the association of preterm delivery with fewer prenatal visits may appear causal, when, in fact, it probably is not.

The second measure, based on the reported date of the first prenatal visit, emphasizes the recommendation that care should begin "early," in the first trimester of pregnancy. Generally, care beginning in the second trimester is referred to as "delayed," and care deferred until the last trimester is termed "late." Although this measure overcomes some of the problems that the frequency index presents, it does not address the fact that early care does not necessarily mean continuous care. For example, a woman may register early in pregnancy to help arrange hospitalization for delivery but not appear again until the third trimester. Despite this shortcoming, the time-of-onset measure is commonly used because the data needed to compute it are widely available.

---

*The 1989 revision of the U.S. Standard Certificate of Live Birth, overseen by the National Center for Health Statistics, recommends several changes that, if adopted by all states, should improve analyses of the use and effectiveness of prenatal care and of interstate differences.

The third method, primarily the Kessner index, provides a more precise, multidimensional measure of prenatal care; however, it is complicated to compute, and for many births data are lacking on one or more of the three variables that make up the index (month in which prenatal care was begun, number of visits, and gestational age). A number of modified versions of the Kessner index have been proposed, including one by Kotelchuck.[8]

The measure used most often in this volume is the trimester in which prenatal care was begun, using the terms "early, delayed, and late," as just defined. The terms "adequate, intermediate, and inadequate" are Kessner index phrases, also defined above. The term "insufficient" is used as a general description of care that is neither adequate nor initiated early in pregnancy; similarly, "sufficient" is used as a general label to describe care that begins early in pregnancy and is sustained until delivery.

A final point: Where vital statistics data are used in this chapter, the data technically refer to infants rather than mothers, because each record is based on an individual birth certificate. However, since multiple births are relatively infrequent (21 per 1,000 live births in 1985) and few women have more than one birth in any year, the terms "women," "mothers," and "births" are often used interchangeably.

CURRENT PATTERNS OF USE*

According to 1985 birth certificate data for the 50 states and the District of Columbia, 76.2 percent of all infants were born to women who obtained early prenatal care, 18.1 percent to women who delayed care, 4.0 percent to women who obtained care late, and 1.7 percent to mothers who had no prenatal care at all (Table 1.1). In absolute numbers, of the approximately 3.8 million babies born in the United States in 1985, about 2.8 million were born to women who began prenatal care early in pregnancy, about 663,000 to women who delayed care, some 150,000 to women who obtained care late, and about 61,000 to women who had no prenatal care at all (Table 1.2).

When vital statistics are analyzed to determine rates of adequate care rather than trimester of onset, a slightly different picture emerges. Hughes et al. found that in 1985 only 68.2 percent of all women obtained adequate care, 23.9 percent had an intermediate level of care, and 7.9 percent of all women had inadequate care.[9]

The following sections describe women's use of prenatal care as measured by six sociodemographic factors: race or ethnic origin, age, education, birth order, marital status, and income.

---

*All data in this section are vital statistics compiled by the National Center for Health Statistics, unless otherwise noted.

TABLE 1.1   Month of Pregnancy in Which Prenatal Care Was Begun (Percent), by Age and Race, United States, 1985

	Month Care Begun (%)			
Age	1–3	4–6	7–9	None
White				
Under 15	38.3	39.8	15.1	6.9
15–19	56.8	32.3	8.0	2.9
20–24	74.7	19.3	4.3	1.6
25–29	85.5	11.4	2.2	0.9
30–34	87.5	9.9	1.8	0.7
35–39	84.5	12.0	2.4	1.1
40+	75.1	18.2	4.5	2.2
Total	79.4	15.8	3.4	1.3
Black				
Under 15	34.4	46.1	13.6	5.9
15–19	47.3	38.3	10.0	4.4
20–24	60.1	29.3	7.1	3.5
25–29	70.3	22.3	4.7	2.7
30–34	73.2	20.1	4.1	2.6
35–39	71.2	21.5	4.4	3.0
40+	63.5	26.8	5.7	4.0
Total	61.8	28.2	6.7	3.4
All Races				
Under 15	36.0	43.5	14.2	6.3
15–19	53.9	34.1	8.6	3.4
20–24	71.7	21.4	4.9	2.0
25–29	83.1	13.1	2.6	1.1
30–34	85.5	11.4	2.2	1.0
35–39	82.4	13.4	2.8	1.3
40+	72.9	19.8	4.8	2.5
Total	76.2	18.1	4.0	1.7

SOURCE: National Center for Health Statistics. Advance report of final natality statistics, 1985. Monthly Vital Statistics Report, Vol. 36, No. 4 Suppl. DHHS Pub. No. (PHS)87-1120. Hyattsville, Md., 1987.

Racial and Ethnic Subgroups

Racial disparities in the use of prenatal care are substantial (Table 1.1). In 1985, black women were far less likely than white women to begin care early and twice as likely to receive late or no care. In absolute numbers, almost 140,000 white infants and almost 60,000 black infants were born to women who had late or no prenatal care (Table 1.2). The higher rates of late or no care among black women are probably due to the greater concentration in this population of several risk factors associated with insufficient prenatal care: limited education, being unmarried (in 1985, 11 percent of white births were to unmarried women versus 57 percent of black births), and, in particular, poverty.

TABLE 1.2   Month of Pregnancy in Which Prenatal Care Was Begun (Number), by Age and Race, United States, 1985

Age	Month Care Begun (no.)				Total (no.)	Unknown (no.)
	1–3	4–6	7–9	None		
White						
Under 15	1,511	1,569	595	272	4,101	154
15–19	176,527	100,276	24,755	9,130	318,725	8,037
20–24	654,059	169,405	37,860	14,393	894,195	18,478
25–29	836,861	112,063	21,594	8,539	997,233	18,176
30–34	498,630	56,642	10,345	4,125	580,398	10,656
35–39	143,587	20,364	4,153	1,868	173,681	3,709
40+	16,853	4,089	999	493	23,040	606
Total	2,328,028	464,408	100,301	38,820	2,991,373	59,816
Black						
Under 15	1,947	2,607	767	335	5,860	204
15–19	61,324	49,716	12,909	5,722	134,270	4,599
20–24	120,704	58,862	14,197	6,988	207,330	6,579
25–29	103,869	32,851	6,974	3,960	152,306	4,652
30–34	55,355	15,176	3,094	1,967	78,129	2,537
35–39	17,986	5,438	1,098	746	26,216	948
40+	2,495	1,053	224	157	4,082	153
Total	363,680	165,703	39,263	19,875	608,193	19,672
All Races						
Under 15	3,547	4,283	1,398	623	10,220	369
15–19	244,723	155,073	39,129	15,364	467,485	13,196
20–24	799,206	238,463	54,921	22,197	1,141,320	26,533
25–29	978,340	154,195	31,061	13,202	1,201,350	24,552
30–34	582,791	77,647	14,913	6,549	696,354	14,454
35–39	172,441	28,120	5,826	2,814	214,336	5,135
40+	20,849	5,669	1,367	718	29,496	893
Total	2,801,897	663,450	148,615	61,467	3,760,561	85,132

SOURCE: National Center for Health Statistics. Advance report of final natality statistics, 1985. Monthly Vital Statistics Report, Vol. 36, No. 4 Suppl. DHHS Pub. No. (PHS)87-1120. Hyattsville, Md., 1987.

TABLE 1.3   Percentage of Babies Born to Women Obtaining Early and
Late or No Care, by Hispanic and Non-Hispanic Origin, Various
Reporting Areas, 1978, 1982, and 1985

| Care Received | | Hispanic | | | | | Non-Hispanic | | |
	Mexican	Puerto Rican	Cuban	Central and South American	Other	Total	White	Black	Total
				1978[a]					
Early	58.7	47.7	75.9	51.5	67.0	57.0	80.7	59.1	77.0
Late or none	11.5	19.9	6.5	16.0	8.3	13.1	3.3	10.9	4.6
				1982[b]					
Early	60.7	54.5	79.3	58.5	66.0	61.0	81.2	60.1	76.9
Late or none	12.0	17.2	4.9	13.4	9.3	12.1	3.8	10.5	5.2
				1985[c]					
Early	60.0	58.3	82.5	60.6	65.8	61.2	81.5	60.5	77.1
Late or none	12.9	15.5	3.7	12.5	9.4	12.4	4.0	10.7	5.4

SOURCES:
[a]National Center for Health Statistics. Births of Hispanic parentage, 1978. Prepared
by Ventura SJ and Heuser RL. Monthly Vital Statistics Report, Vol. 29, No. 12 Suppl.
DHHS Pub. No. (PHS)81-1120. Hyattsville, Md., 1981 (17 states and the District of
Columbia reporting).
[b]National Center for Health Statistics. Births of Hispanic parentage, 1982. Prepared
by Ventura SJ. Monthly Vital Statistics Report, Vol. 34, No. 4 Suppl. DHHS Pub. No.
(PHS)85-1120. Hyattsville, Md., 1985 (23 states and the District of Columbia
reporting).
[c]National Center for Health Statistics. Births of Hispanic parentage, 1985. Prepared
by Ventura SJ and Heuser RL. Monthly Vital Statistics Report, Vol. 36, No. 11 Suppl.
DHHS Pub. No. (PHS)88-1120. Hyattsville, Md., 1988 (23 states and the District of
Columbia reporting).

Use of prenatal care by mothers of Hispanic origin has been analyzed for
the District of Columbia and the 23 states that routinely collect information on Hispanic births. More than 92 percent of the total U.S. Hispanic
population lived in these jurisdictions in 1985, and over 370,000 births to
mothers of Hispanic origin were reported. Of these births, the vast majority
(95 percent) were listed as being of white race on the birth certificate,
two-thirds were to women of Mexican origin, and nearly half (47 percent)
were to mothers who had been born in the United States.[10]

Generally, Hispanic mothers are substantially less likely than non-
Hispanic white mothers to begin prenatal care early and are three times as
likely to obtain late or no care. Moreover, as Table 1.3 shows, Hispanic
mothers as a group are more likely than non-Hispanic black mothers to

TABLE 1.4   Percentage of Babies Born to Women Obtaining Early and Late or No Care, for Asian or Pacific Islander, American Indian, White, and Black Subgroups and for All Races, United States, 1985

Care Received	Asian or Pacific Islander						American Indian	White	Black	All Races
	Chinese	Japanese	Hawaiian	Filipino	Other	Total				
Early	82.3	85.8	70.6	77.2	70.7	75.0	60.3	79.4	61.8	76.2
Late or none	4.2	2.7	6.5	4.6	7.8	6.2	11.5	4.7	10.1	5.7

SOURCE: Unpublished vital statistics data from the National Center for Health Statistics.

begin care late or not at all.* Interestingly, mothers of Cuban background are an anomaly among Hispanic women in their use of prenatal services. They were even more likely than non-Hispanic white mothers to begin prenatal care early in pregnancy, and only 3.7 percent of Cuban mothers in 1985 had late or no care. Such subgroup diversity suggests that the problem of inadequate care among Hispanic women is not due to Hispanic origin per se, but rather to other factors—probably income, education, previous experiences with other health care systems, or a combination of the three.

Other major U.S. subgroups whose use of prenatal care has been analyzed include American Indian (not including native Alaskans) and Asian or Pacific Islander women (Table 1.4). Out of 3.8 million births in the United States in 1985, there were about 41,000 to American Indians and 112,000 to Asian or Pacific Islander women. In that same year, Chinese, Japanese, and Filipino women exhibited particularly high rates of participation in care and were less likely than white women to obtain late or no care; Hawaiian women and other subgroups of women in this category (including Indian, Cambodian, Laotian, Vietnamese, Korean, and other Asian or Pacific Islander women) placed between white and black women in the late or no-care category. American Indian women, however, were more likely than either white or black women to obtain late or no care.

Use of prenatal care also varies with a pregnant woman's place of birth. For example, two studies of prenatal care use among selected groups in New York City found that recent immigrants were less likely to obtain late

---

*Although Table 1.3 and some others that follow present data for several years in addition to 1985, discussion of trends does not begin until later in this chapter. Here, the focus is on 1985 patterns of use only.

or no care than women born in the United States.[11,12] By contrast, a large
follow-back survey of 1986 births in Massachusetts found that foreign-
born women were more likely to obtain late or no care than U.S.-born
women (24 percent versus 37 percent, respectively).[13] Differences in local
health care systems, in the magnitude of language barriers, and in the
immigrant populations themselves may account for such variation. Most
experts in maternity services believe that recently arrived immigrants are
at high risk of obtaining insufficient prenatal care.

Age

Timing of entry into prenatal care also varies with the age of the mother
(Table 1.1). In general, young mothers are at high risk of obtaining late or
no prenatal care, with the greatest risk for the youngest mothers.[14]
Adolescent mothers are the age group least likely to obtain early prenatal
care and most likely to begin care late or not at all, but there are some
interesting variations in utilization between black and white teenage
mothers, as shown in Table 1.1. Although white mothers under 15 are
slightly more likely than black mothers under 15 to begin prenatal care in
the first trimester, they are also more likely to begin care in the third
trimester or not at all. The number of births to these very young women,
however, is small—10,220 in 1985.

Use of prenatal care among teenagers has also been analyzed using the
more refined measure of adequacy. Examining the adequacy of care is
particularly appropriate for this group, because teenagers may be more
likely than older women to participate in care episodically. Using 1980
National Natality Survey data, one study found that mothers under age 20
were nearly twice as likely to have inadequate care as mothers age 20 to 24
(16.4 and 8.4 percent, respectively).[15]

Older mothers, much as teenagers, tend to delay entry into prenatal care
(Table 1.1). Mothers age 40 and over are less likely than mothers age 25
to 39 to begin care in the first trimester and more likely to obtain care late
or not at all. This tendency increases as women get older, and women over
age 45 become as likely as or more likely than mothers age 15 to 19 to
obtain late or no care.[16] As for very young teenagers, however, the number
of births to older mothers is small—fewer than 30,000 to women age 40 or
above in 1985.

Education

Timing of the first prenatal visit correlates highly with level of education. In 1985, 88 percent of mothers with at least some college education
began care early in pregnancy, compared with 58 percent of mothers who

TABLE 1.5 Percentage of Babies Born to Women Obtaining Late or No Care, by Race and Education, United States, 1975, 1980, and 1985

Years of Education	1985[a]	1980[a]	1975[b]
	White		
0–8	14.4	13.4	13.6
9–11	9.6	8.5	8.6
12	3.5	2.9	3.2
13+	1.5	1.4	1.6
Total	4.0	3.8	4.2
	Black		
0–8	15.7	15.2	15.8
9–11	14.4	12.6	13.3
12	9.3	7.7	9.3
13+	4.9	4.5	5.8
Total	10.1	9.0	10.9
	All Races		
0–8	14.7	14.1	14.4
9–11	11.2	9.8	10.2
12	4.6	3.8	4.2
13+	2.0	1.9	2.1
Total	5.3	4.8	5.7

SOURCES:
[a]Published and unpublished vital statistics data from the National Center for Health Statistics.
[b]National Center for Health Statistics. Prenatal care, United States, 1969–75. Prepared by Taffel SM. Vital and Health Statistics, Series 21, No. 33. DHEW Pub. No. (PHS)78-1911. Washington, D.C.: Government Printing Office, 1978.

had less than a high school education.[17] Similarly, the probability that a pregnant woman will obtain care late or not at all decreases steadily as her educational level increases (Table 1.5).

Given the strong association between higher levels of education and early enrollment in prenatal care, it is useful to consider the proportion of mothers in various subpopulations who have completed high school. In both 1984 and 1985, 79 percent of all mothers had completed at least 12 years of schooling—82 percent of white mothers, 68 percent of black mothers.[18] In 1984, more than twice the proportion of Native American mothers (American Indians and Native Alaskans) as white mothers had less than 12 years of education (38 percent versus 18 percent). Native American mothers were also more likely than black mothers not to have

TABLE 1.6   Percentage of Babies Born to Women Obtaining Late or No
Care, by Birth Order and Race, Reporting Areas, 1975, 1980, and 1985

Birth Order	1985[a]	1980[a]	1975[b]
	White		
First	4.1	3.8	4.8
Second	4.0	3.5	3.9
Third	5.4	4.5	4.9
Fourth	7.8	6.6	7.0
Fifth+	13.1	11.3	12.6
	Black		
First	8.8	7.8	9.6
Second	9.4	8.4	10.2
Third	10.6	9.0	10.6
Fourth	12.9	10.6	11.7
Fifth+	16.5	13.5	13.9
	All Races		
First	4.9	4.6	5.6
Second	4.8	4.4	4.9
Third	6.4	5.5	6.0
Fourth	9.1	7.7	8.1
Fifth+	14.2	12.8	13.2

SOURCES:
[a]Published and unpublished vital statistics data from the National Center for Health
Statistics.
[b]National Center for Health Statistics. Prenatal care, United States, 1969–75.
Prepared by Taffel SM. Vital and Health Statistics, Series 21, No. 33. DHEW Pub. No.
(PHS)78-1911. Washington, D.C.: Government Printing Office, 1978.

completed high school.[19] For mothers of Hispanic origin, 21 states (not
including California and Texas) reported in 1984 on educational attainment;
overall, 45 percent of Hispanic mothers giving birth in that year had not
completed at least 12 years of school, with subgroup proportions ranging
from 59 percent for Mexican mothers to 22 percent for Cuban mothers.[20]

Birth Order

Obtaining late or no prenatal care is also associated with birth order. In
general, the more children a woman has had, the more likely she is to delay
care or to seek none at all. In 1985, close to 5 percent of both first and
second children were born to mothers who obtained late or no care (Table
1.6). About 6 percent of third births fell into this category, however, and
the numbers increased to 9 and 14 percent for fourth and fifth children,

respectively. The association of delayed care with greater numbers of children is reflected in the prenatal care use of older mothers: in 1985, nearly 60 percent of births to mothers over age 45 were fifth or subsequent children.[21]

The relationship of prenatal care to birth order varies slightly with race. For white mothers, the percentage of infants born with late or no care is lowest for second births; that number increases steadily with subsequent births. For black mothers, first births are the least likely to have had late or no prenatal care; the risk increases with each subsequent birth. Taffel has concluded that the different age distribution of white and black women at the time of first birth explains these minor variations.[22]

Marital Status

Pregnant women who are married are more likely to obtain sufficient prenatal care than pregnant women who are not married (Table 1.7). This relationship holds true among women within the same racial or ethnic group and with similar levels of education.[23] Unmarried mothers are more than three times as likely as married mothers to obtain late or no prenatal

TABLE 1.7 Percentage of Babies Born to Women Obtaining Late or No Care, by Race and Marital Status, United States, 1975, 1980, and 1985

Marital Status	1985[a]	1980[a]	1975[b]
	White		
Married	3.4	3.2	3.9
Unmarried	13.0	13.4	18.9
Total	4.7	4.2	4.9
	Black		
Married	6.0	5.7	7.5
Unmarried	12.8	11.3	13.6
Total	10.0	8.8	10.4
	All Races		
Married	3.4	3.5	4.4
Unmarried	13.0	12.5	16.2
Total	5.7	5.1	6.1

SOURCES:
[a]Published and unpublished vital statistics data from the National Center for Health Statistics.
[b]National Center for Health Statistics. Prenatal care, United States, 1969–75. Prepared by Taffel SM. Vital and Health Statistics, Series 21, No. 33. DHEW Pub. No. (PHS)78-1911. Washington, D.C.: Government Printing Office, 1978.

care. Unmarried white mothers are almost four times as likely as married white mothers to obtain late or no care; and unmarried black mothers are twice as likely as married black mothers to obtain late or no care. Among unmarried mothers, women of Hispanic origin are most likely to obtain late or no care, followed by white non-Hispanic and then black non-Hispanic mothers.

The correlation of unmarried status with insufficient prenatal care has become more important in recent years as childbearing among unmarried women has increased, reaching an all-time high of 828,000 births (about 22 percent of all births) in 1985.[24] In that year, 12 percent of non-Hispanic white births were to unmarried women, compared with 61 percent of non-Hispanic black births and 23 percent of Hispanic births. The range among the latter group, however, is striking: 51 percent of Puerto Rican births were to unmarried women versus 26 percent of Mexican births.[25]

The differential between married and unmarried women's timing of entry into prenatal care lessens somewhat with increasing age; however, at any age unmarried women are much more likely than married women to obtain late or no care.[26] With regard to the relationship among marital status, age, and use of prenatal care, Ventura and Hendershot analyzed 1980 National Natality Survey data and found that "teenage mothers began prenatal care earlier if they were married at conception than if they were not . . . and those who were married after conception but before delivery began prenatal care earlier than those who were not married at the time of delivery. The differences [were] substantial."[27]

Income

Data on the relationship of income to prenatal care use are available from the 1980 National Natality Survey (NNS)[28] and the 1982 National Survey of Family Growth (NSFG).[29] Extensive analysis of NNS data by Singh et al. has yielded the following findings: only 66 percent of women with incomes less than 150 percent of the federal poverty level initiated prenatal care in the first trimester, compared with 85 percent of women with incomes equal to or greater than 250 percent of the poverty level; women with incomes below 150 percent of the poverty level were almost three times as likely as women with incomes equal to or above 250 percent of the poverty level to obtain late or no care; and poor non-Hispanic black and poor non-Hispanic white mothers (again, poverty being income less than 150 percent of the poverty level) were equally likely to obtain inadequate care.[30] Similarly, an analysis of NSFG data found that only 50.4 percent of mothers living below the federal poverty level, as compared with 73.6 percent of nonpoor mothers, began care in the first trimester of pregnancy.[31]

The Massachusetts follow-back study of 1985 births, referred to earlier, also found that the probability of obtaining adequate care increases as income grows. Thirty-eight percent of women with annual incomes of less than $10,000 obtained adequate prenatal care; 64 percent of women with annual incomes between $10,000 and $20,000 were in the adequate care category; and for women with annual incomes between $40,000 and $50,000, the percentage climbed to 88.[32]

Given that one-third of all U.S. births are to women with incomes less than 150 percent of the federal poverty level,[33] the consistent correlation of low income with insufficient prenatal care is of major importance and forms the basis of many recommendations that appear later in this report.

RELATIONSHIPS AMONG DEMOGRAPHIC RISK FACTORS

To assess the comparative importance of selected demographic factors in predicting use of prenatal care, Singh et al. constructed estimates of relative risk for late or no prenatal care for various groups.[34] In this analysis, 17 populations (including the total U.S. population) are compared with the group in the United States that has the best rates of prenatal care utilization—married, white, nonpoor women. The question is posed: Compared with the reference group, how many times more likely is group X to obtain late or no prenatal care? As shown in Table 1.8, unmarried women had the greatest relative risk of late or no care. Teenagers, women with less than a high school education, Hispanic women, and women with incomes less than 150 percent of the federal poverty level also faced substantially greater risks.

Some investigators have cross-tabulated use of prenatal care with combinations of three or more demographic measures. Such analyses help in understanding the interaction among risk factors and in pinpointing populations at high risk of insufficient prenatal care. Ingram et al., for example, showed that in 1983 only about 45 percent of unmarried teenagers with less than a high school education obtained early prenatal care (44.1 percent of black teenagers and 46.3 percent of white teenagers). Conversely, about 85 percent of married women age 20 and older with more than a high school education obtained early care (81.9 percent of black women and 90.7 of white women). Generally, this pattern also held true for late or no care.[35]

Table 1.9 reveals that the impact of poverty on use of prenatal care varies with marital status and that the magnitude of these relationships, in turn, varies with age, race, education, and place of residence. This table underscores the high risk of inadequate prenatal care among poor women who are unmarried, particularly those who are young, not well educated, living in rural areas, or Hispanic.

Chapter 3 summarizes several multivariate analyses that consider the relative importance of numerous factors that increase the risk of insufficient prenatal care. The demographic measures discussed in this chapter appear in many of those analyses.

TABLE 1.8   Number of Mothers Obtaining Late or No Prenatal Care and Relative Risk, Reference Group, Selected Subgroups, and Total Population, United States, 1980

Subgroup	Number (thousands)	Relative Risk
Reference group—married, white, nonpoor[a]	—	1.0[b]
Age		
<20	55	4.3
20–24	61	2.0
≥25	53	1.3
Race/ethnic origin		
Black (non-Hispanic)	39	3.1
White (non-Hispanic)	104	1.6
Hispanic	26	4.0
Marital status		
Married	90	1.4
Unmarried	79	5.1
Residence		
Metropolitan	108	2.0
Nonmetropolitan	61	2.2
Education (years)		
<12	77	4.0
12	65	1.7
≥13	27	1.0
Income (% of poverty level)		
<150	100	3.7
150–249	22	1.1
≥250	47	1.3
Total	169	2.0

[a]An income of 150 percent of the poverty level or more is considered nonpoor.

[b]Risk of 1.0 for the reference group represents a level of inadequate care of 2 percent (with inadequate care defined as care in the third trimester or no care). For each other subgroup, risk is computed by dividing the proportion in that subgroup receiving inadequate care by the proportion in the reference group receiving comparable care.

SOURCE: Singh S, Torres D, and Forrest JD. The need for prenatal care in the United States: Evidence from the 1980 National Natality Survey. Fam. Plan. Perspect. 17:122–123, 1985, tables 5 and 6. Reprinted with permission of the Alan Guttmacher Institute.

TABLE 1.9 Percentage of Mothers in Selected Subgroups Obtaining Inadequate Prenatal Care, by Income and Marital Status[a]

Subgroup	Poor (<150% of poverty level)		Nonpoor (≥150% of poverty level)	
	Married	Unmarried	Married	Unmarried
Age				
<20	5.7	16.4	4.6	11.4
20–24	5.9 }	11.3	2.5 }	6.4
≥25	4.9 }		2.0 }	
Race/ethnic origin				
Black (non-Hispanic)	4.9	12.3	2.9	3.8
White (non-Hispanic)	5.1	(12.0)	2.2	(12.8)
Hispanic	8.3	(25.4)	4.5	(3.4)
Residence				
Metropolitan	5.5	12.5	2.1	8.4
Nonmetropolitan	5.3	(16.7)	2.8	(6.4)
Education (years)				
<12	8.6	16.5	4.9	3.9
12	4.9 }	(9.9)	2.0 }	(9.6)
≥13	0.8 }		1.9 }	
Total	5.4	13.6	2.3	7.9

[a]Data for married women are from the 1980 National Natality Survey (NNS). For unmarried women, estimates (given in parentheses) have been computed by applying poverty status distributions from the 1982 National Survey of Family Growth (NSFG) (among women grouped by trimester of care) to the numbers of unmarried women in the NNS receiving adequate and inadequate care. Because the NSFG sample of births to unmarried women is small, and the number of unmarried women in the NNS within subgroups is often extremely small, the resulting estimates for poor, unmarried women are sometimes unstable. Some subgroups have been combined because of the very small numbers of cases. Differences between poor and nonpoor women are statistically significant at $p < .05$, using the two-tailed t test, except among the following subgroups: married women—teenagers, blacks, Hispanics, and women with ≥13 years of education; unmarried women—whites and women with ≥12 years of education.

SOURCE: Singh S, Torres D, and Forrest JD. The need for prenatal care in the United States: Evidence from the 1980 National Natality Survey. Fam. Plan. Perspect. 17:118, 1985, table 4. Reprinted with permission of the Alan Guttmacher Institute.

GEOGRAPHIC POCKETS OF NEED

Insufficient prenatal care is concentrated in certain geographic areas, just as it is in certain demographic groups. Analyses of 1985 vital statistics data conducted by the Children's Defense Fund found wide disparities among states in the percentage of infants born to women obtaining late or no care (Table 1.10 and Figure 1.1). For example, a woman giving birth

TABLE 1.10   Percentage of Babies Born to Women Obtaining Late or No Care, All Races, All States and the District of Columbia, 1969, 1975, 1979, and 1985

State	1985^a	1979^a	1975^b	1969^b
Alabama	6.2	6.3	—	—
Alaska	4.4	5.1	—	—
Arizona	7.7	8.1	13.5	20.9
Arkansas	7.4	6.3	—	—
California	5.4	4.9	6.0	7.2
Colorado	5.4	4.7	5.2	—
Connecticut	3.0	2.3	2.6	—
Delaware	4.3	4.5	3.9	—
District of Columbia	11.4	8.0	14.8	22.8
Florida	9.0	7.0	7.8	—
Georgia	5.3	6.0	7.5	—
Hawaii	5.1	4.9	5.5	7.4
Idaho	5.4	5.0	—	—
Illinois	4.5	5.2	6.0	8.0
Indiana	5.1	3.9	4.1	6.2
Iowa	2.1	2.3	2.4	3.5
Kansas	3.9	3.4	4.0	5.1
Kentucky	5.1	7.5	6.7	10.2
Louisiana	4.9	5.0	5.9	9.1
Maine	3.5	2.3	3.0	5.2
Maryland	4.1	3.6	3.6	6.7
Massachusetts	2.6	1.6	—	3.8
Michigan	2.9	3.3	4.0	5.4
Minnesota	3.9	3.3	4.2	7.6
Mississippi	4.3	4.5	6.6	11.2
Missouri	4.0	4.0	5.5	8.2
Montana	4.1	3.6	4.4	6.7
Nebraska	3.4	3.4	4.1	6.6
Nevada	6.0	7.2	7.4	7.7
New Hampshire	2.4	2.3	2.8	4.9
New Jersey	4.2	5.1	5.9	9.7
New Mexico	13.4	0.0	—	—
New York	8.9	8.9	8.3	11.1
North Carolina	4.2	4.2	5.0	7.5
North Dakota	2.5	3.3	5.0	7.1
Ohio	3.4	3.3	3.5	5.0
Oklahoma	7.3	8.6	8.2	8.0
Oregon	5.6	4.6	4.9	—
Pennsylvania	4.9	3.9	—	—
Rhode Island	2.3	1.7	1.9	3.8
South Carolina	8.0	6.0	6.7	8.1
South Dakota	5.6	6.5	8.1	10.8

TABLE 1.10 *Continued*

State	1985[a]	1979[a]	1975[b]	1969[b]
Tennessee	5.5	5.3	6.8	11.1
Texas	11.0	8.1	9.4	13.1
Utah	3.1	2.6	2.0	3.8
Vermont	3.5	3.4	4.8	7.0
Virginia	4.0	3.4	—	—
Washington	4.7	3.6	3.8	4.7
West Virginia	6.1	6.3	8.8	11.5
Wisconsin	3.0	2.7	2.6	4.6
Wyoming	4.3	4.7	5.1	7.1
Total	5.7	5.1	6.0	8.2

SOURCES:
[a]Hughes D, Johnson K, Rosenbaum S, Simons J, and Butler E. The Health of America's Children: Maternal and Child Health Data Book. Washington, D.C.: Children's Defense Fund, 1988.
[b]National Center for Health Statistics. Prenatal care, United States, 1969–75. Prepared by Taffel SM. Vital and Health Statistics, Series 21, No. 33. DHEW Pub. No. (PHS)78-1911. Washington, D.C.: Government Printing Office, 1978.

in New York in 1985 was roughly three times as likely as a woman in Michigan or Connecticut to obtain late or no care, and a nonwhite woman in New Mexico or New York was three times as likely as a nonwhite woman in Massachusetts to obtain late or no prenatal care. The analyses also show that states with low percentages of mothers obtaining early care also tend to have high percentages of mothers obtaining late or no prenatal care. In 1985, the three jurisdictions with the lowest percentages of women obtaining early prenatal care and the highest percentages of women with late or no care were New Mexico, the District of Columbia, and Texas.[36]

Even greater variations in levels of prenatal care can exist within states. For example, although New York State as a whole reports that 9 percent of pregnant women in 1985 had late or no prenatal care (Table 1.10), the percentage was about 18 percent in New York City and far higher in some neighborhoods: in the Mott Haven district of the Bronx, more than 50 percent of births in 1985 were to women with no care or care that began in the third trimester.[37]

Public health authorities and health planners have long recognized that certain communities show particularly poor rates of prenatal care use, and many of the recent state and local initiatives to combat infant mortality (see Appendix A) have included careful "mapping" of areas where inadequate use is prevalent. The maps in Figures 1.2 to 1.5 show rates of insufficient prenatal care for various geographic areas. Figures 1.2 and 1.3 are of Wisconsin and

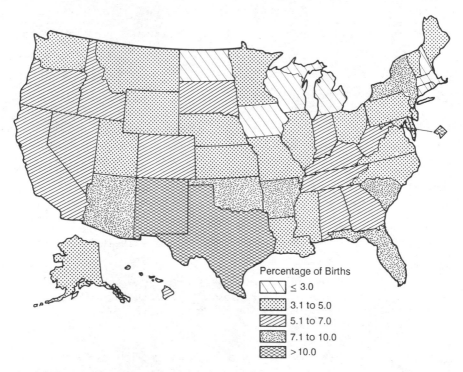

FIGURE 1.1   Percentage of births to women obtaining late or no prenatal care, United States, all races, 1985. SOURCE: Children's Defense Fund.

North Carolina and display, respectively, patterns of late or no care and patterns of inadequate care in 1985. These maps reveal that rural as well as urban areas exhibit pockets of insufficient prenatal care. Figures 1.4 and 1.5 present a 1985 geographic profile of late or no registration in prenatal care for the District of Columbia and New Haven, Connecticut. Although each of these maps takes a somewhat idiosyncratic approach to defining and displaying geographic variations in use of prenatal care, they effectively communicate the simple fact that pockets of need exist and can be pinpointed. Such maps also show that aggregate data, both state and national, can obscure the fact that use of prenatal care can be exceedingly poor in some smaller areas.

These geographic "hot spots" are perhaps best explained by variations in income levels within states and communities. As noted earlier, low income is among the most important factors explaining insufficient use of prenatal care. Thus, census tracts with high concentrations of low-income individuals are likely to have high rates of insufficient prenatal care. Other factors that probably account for these geographic

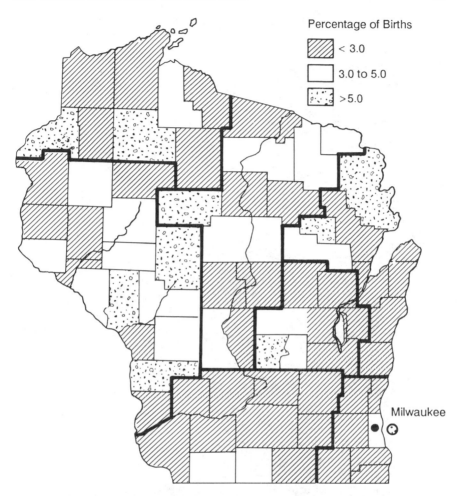

FIGURE 1.2 Percentage of births to women obtaining late or no prenatal care, Wisconsin, by county, all races, 1985. SOURCE: Wisconsin Department of Health and Social Services.

concentrations of need include local inadequacies in the health care system and transportation problems. These obstacles to care and others are taken up in Chapter 2.

TRENDS IN THE USE OF PRENATAL CARE

Several special studies[38–42] combined with U.S. natality statistics published by the National Center for Health Statistics,[43] make possible an

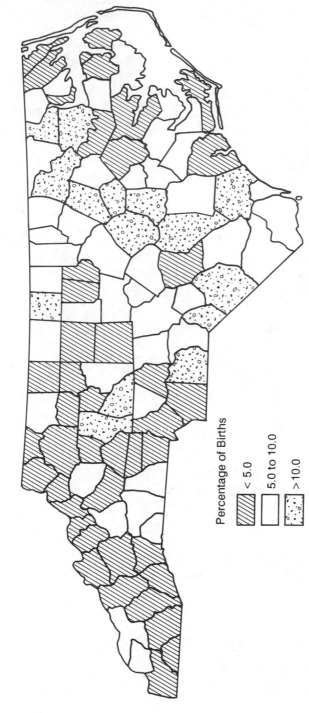

FIGURE 1.3 Percentage of births to women obtaining inadequate care, North Carolina, by county, all races, 1985. Inadequate care is care beginning in the third trimester or four or fewer visits for a pregnancy of 34 or more weeks (Kessner). SOURCE: North Carolina State Center for Health Statistics.

Percentage of Births

< 5.0

5.0 to 10.0

>10.0

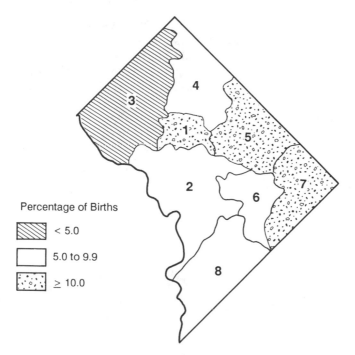

Percentage of Births

        < 5.0

        5.0 to 9.9

        ≥ 10.0

FIGURE 1.4   Percentage of births to women obtaining late or no prenatal care, District of Columbia, by ward, 1985. SOURCE: D.C. Department of Human Services.

analysis of trends in the use of prenatal care from 1969 to 1985. Table 1.11 shows steady improvement from 1969 through 1980 in the percentage of births to mothers receiving prenatal care in the first trimester of pregnancy. Since 1980, however, this percentage has remained stable or decreased. Among black women, declines in early use of prenatal care were registered in 1981, 1982, and 1985.

Table 1.12, which displays rates of late or no care, reveals a particularly troubling trend. There has apparently been an increase since 1980 in the percentage of births to women with late or no prenatal care. Although this trend applies to all races, the increase is more pronounced among black women. In 1981, 8.8 percent of births to black women were in this category; by 1985, 10 percent were. In fact, 1985 rates of late or no prenatal care for black women are about the same as those recorded in 1976; improvements in the interim have, in effect, been erased. An analysis of trends in the use of prenatal care between 1970 and 1983 found that early enrollment for black mothers in 1982 was 3.6 percentage points below what it would have been if the 1976 to 1980 trend had continued, and 10.8 percentage points below the expected level based on the 1970 to 1975 trend.[44]

Given the size and diversity of this country, it is important to consider whether all states mirror these national trends or whether a few states are responsible for observed changes. Table 1.10 shows use of prenatal care for selected years from 1969 to 1985, based on national data for all 50 states and the District of Columbia. (Although 1969 data are not available from 13 states and in 1975 8 states had not yet begun to collect data on time of entry into prenatal care, general state trends can nonetheless be seen.)

There was a clear pattern of improved use of prenatal care on the state level in the early 1970s. All 37 reporting states and the District of Columbia showed smaller percentages of women obtaining late or no care in 1975, as compared to 1969. Most states demonstrated decreases of

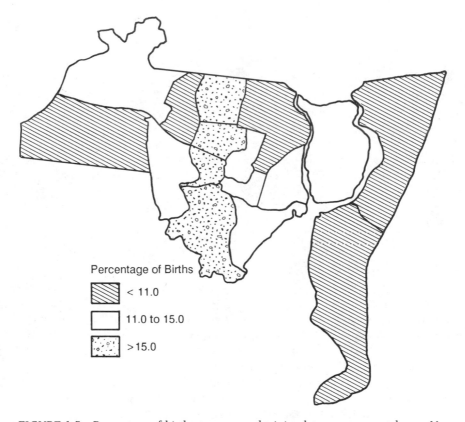

Percentage of Births

⬚ < 11.0

⬚ 11.0 to 15.0

⬚ > 15.0

FIGURE 1.5   Percentage of births to women obtaining late or no prenatal care, New Haven, Connecticut, by neighborhood, all races, 1982–1985. SOURCE: de Andres P, Backus L, Greene M, Pope E, Scholle R, Singleton C, and Triffin E. Targeting the Problems behind New Haven's Infant Mortality Rate. A report of a community project conducted by students at the Department of Epidemiology and Public Health, Yale School of Medicine. New Haven, Ct. Spring 1985.

TABLE 1.11   Percentage of Babies Born to Women Obtaining Early
Care, by Race, United States, 1969–1985

Year	White	Black	Total
1969	72.4	42.7	68.5
1970	72.4	44.3	67.9
1971	73.0	46.6	68.6
1972	73.6	49.0	69.4
1973	74.9	51.4	70.8
1974	75.9	53.9	72.1
1975	75.9	55.8	72.3
1976	76.8	57.7	73.5
1977	77.3	59.0	74.1
1978	78.2	60.2	74.9
1979	79.1	61.6	75.9
1980	79.3	62.7	76.3
1981	79.4	62.4	76.3
1982	79.3	61.5	76.1
1983	79.4	61.5	76.2
1984	79.6	62.2	76.5
1985	79.4	61.8	76.2

SOURCE: Published and unpublished vital statistics data from the National Center
for Health Statistics.

between 25 and 30 percent, and late or no care decreased by nearly 40
percent in several states between 1969 and 1975.

These favorable trends continued into the late 1970s. From 1975 to
1979, all but 7 of the 43 reporting jurisdictions showed continued declines
in the percentage of babies born to women who had received late or no
care. However, the rate of decline had slowed, and 6 of the 7 states showed
an increase.

Between 1979 and 1985, the increase in the percentage of women
obtaining late or no care evidenced in national statistics was mirrored in
states from every region of the country. For example, although the number
of women beginning care late or not at all in the District of Columbia
dropped by 65 percent between 1969 and 1979, the number increased 43
percent between 1979 and 1985. In Oregon and Indiana, the percentages
of women who had no prenatal care or none before the seventh month of
pregnancy were greater in 1985 than in any other year since 1975. Maine,
Massachusetts, and Utah are states with generally low percentages of late
or no prenatal care, yet they, too, experienced increases between 1979 and
1985. South Carolina and Florida experienced upward trends of about 30
percent each between 1979 and 1985. Overall, 20 states experienced an
increase in the percentage of women who obtained late or no care during

TABLE 1.12   Percentage of Babies Born to Women Obtaining Late or
No Care, by Race, United States, 1969–1985

Year	White	Black	Total
1969	6.3	18.2	7.3
1970	6.2	16.6	7.9
1971	5.8	14.6	7.2
1972	5.5	13.2	7.0
1973	5.4	12.4	6.7
1974	5.0	11.4	6.2
1975	5.0	10.5	6.0
1976	4.8	9.9	5.7
1977	4.7	9.6	5.6
1978	4.5	9.3	5.4
1979	4.3	8.9	5.1
1980	4.3	8.8	5.1
1981	4.3	9.1	5.2
1982	4.5	9.6	5.5
1983	4.6	9.7	5.6
1984	4.7	9.6	5.6
1985	4.7	10.0	5.7

SOURCE: Published and unpublished vital statistics data from the National Center
for Health Statistics.

this period, and a dozen more states showed no decrease. The Ingram et al.
study of the use of prenatal care between 1970 and 1983 confirms the
finding that the trends observed on the national level reflect changes in
many states from all regions.[45]

It is not known what factors account for these disturbing trends,
although a number of social, economic, and other changes in the 1980s
have been offered as explanations. These include the increase in unemployment in the early 1980s and the resulting loss of employer-based
health insurance and personal income; the increasing proportion of
women of childbearing age living in poverty; and the increasing number of
employed individuals who have inadequate or no health insurance, along
with the continuing erosion of maternity benefits under private plans.
Other reasons include the cutbacks in Medicaid eligibility in the early
1980s and the declining proportion of the poor covered by Medicaid; the
increasing proportion of births to unmarried women and the growth in the
number of households headed by single women; and the increasingly
limited capacity of the health care systems relied on by low-income women
for prenatal care, caused by funding restrictions and the malpractice
squeeze, which is shrinking the pool of obstetric care providers. Many of
these issues are discussed in Chapter 2.

Other important trends between about 1970 and the mid-1980s include the following:

a. The gap between black and white rates of prenatal care use narrowed between 1970 and 1983, although the pace at which it was closing slowed toward the latter half of that interval.[46]

b. Adolescent mothers were more likely to obtain early care in 1985 than they were in 1970. Generally, there has been a decline in late or no care among teenagers; however, the decline has been least for the youngest mothers, and, as among older women, progress has slowed in the 1980's.[47]

c. As for black women, increasing percentages of some subgroups of Hispanic women—particularly Mexican women—obtained late or no care in the 1980s (Table 1.3).

d. In recent years, there has been virtually no improvement in the proportion of women with little education who obtained late or no care (Table 1.5).

e. Between 1970 and 1985, unmarried mothers, particularly unmarried white mothers, exhibited some of the most rapid decreases in late registration for prenatal care (Table 1.7).

f. Data from 1975, 1980, and 1985 consistently show that for black women, first births are the least likely to have had late or no prenatal care; for white women, second births are the least likely to fall in this category (Table 1.6).

SUMMARY

Several interrelated demographic factors put women at risk for insufficient prenatal care: being in a racial or ethnic minority group (especially American Indian, black, and Hispanic), being under 20 (particularly, under 15), having less than a high school education, higher parity, and being unmarried. Geographic analysis also reveals that insufficient use of prenatal care is often concentrated in areas that can be easily identified. All of these risk factors, in turn, are closely related to poverty, which is one of the most important factors consistently associated with insufficient prenatal care.

Unfortunately, the steady progress of the 1970s in drawing more women into prenatal care early in pregnancy ended in the 1980s. On the important measure of late or no care, there has actually been a reversal of progress, particularly for black women.

REFERENCES AND NOTES

1. American College of Obstetricians and Gynecologists. Standards for Obstetric-Gynecologic Services, 6th ed. Washington, D.C., 1985.

2. American Academy of Pediatrics and American College of Obstetricians and Gynecologists. Guidelines for Perinatal Care. Washington, D.C., 1983.
3. Morehead MA, Donaldson RS, and Seravalli MS. Comparisons between OEO Neighborhood Health Centers and other health care providers of ratings of the quality of health care. Am. J. Public Health 61:1294–1306, 1971.
4. Hughey MJ. Routine prenatal and gynecologic care in prepaid group practice. J. Am. Med. Assoc. 256:1775–1777, 1986.
5. Kessner DM, Singer J, Kalk CE, and Schlesinger ER. Infant death: An analysis by maternal risk and health care. In Contrasts in Health Status, Vol. 1. Washington, D.C.: National Academy of Sciences, 1973.
6. National Center for Health Statistics. Comparability of reporting between the birth certificate and the National Natality Survey. Prepared by Querec LJ. Vital and Health Statistics, Series 2, No. 83. DHEW Pub. No. (PHS)80-1357. Washington, D.C.: Government Printing Office, 1980.
7. National Center for Health Statistics. Birth certificate completion procedures and the accuracy of Missouri birth certificate data. Prepared by Land G and Vaughan B. Priorities in Health Statistics: Proceedings of the 19th National Meeting of the Public Health Conference on Records and Statistics, August 1983. DHHS Pub. No. (PHS)81-1214. Washington, D.C.: Government Printing Office, 1983, pp. 263–265.
8. Kotelchuck M. The mismeasurement of prenatal care adequacy in the U.S. and a proposed alternative two-part index. Paper presented at the American Public Health Association annual meeting, New Orleans, 1987.
9. Hughes D, Johnson K, Rosenbaum S, Simons J, and Butler E. The Health of America's Children: Maternal and Child Health Data Book. Washington, D.C.: Children's Defense Fund, 1988. The definition of adequate care used in these analyses differs slightly from that in the Kessner index: gestational age at which measurement begins is 17 weeks in this modified index versus 13 or fewer weeks in the Kessner index.
10. National Center for Health Statistics. Births of Hispanic parentage, 1985. Prepared by Ventura SJ. Monthly Vital Statistics Report, Vol. 36, No. 11 Suppl. DHHS Pub. No. (PHS)88-1120. Hyattsville, Md., 1988.
11. Chao S, Imaizumi S, Gorman S, and Lowenstein R. Reasons for absence of prenatal care and its consequences. New York: Department of Obstetrics and Gynecology, Harlem Hospital Center, 1984.
12. Kalmuss D, Darabi KF, Lopez I, Caro FG, Marshall E, and Carter A. Barriers to Prenatal Care: An Examination of Use of Prenatal Care Among Low-Income Women in New York City. New York: Community Service Society, 1987.
13. Johnson S, Gibbs E, Kogan M, Kapp C, and Hansen JH. Massachusetts Prenatal Care Survey—Factors Related to Prenatal Care Utilization. Boston: SPRANS Prenatal Care Project, Massachusetts Department of Public Health, 1987.
14. Hughes D et al. Op. cit., p. 29.
15. The Financing of Maternity Care in the United States. New York: Alan Guttmacher Institute, 1987, p. 45.
16. National Center for Health Statistics, Division of Vital Statistics. Unpublished data, 1984.
17. National Center for Health Statistics. Advance report of final natality statistics, 1985. Monthly Vital Statistics Report, Vol. 36, No. 4 Suppl. DHHS Pub. No. (PHS)87-1120. Hyattsville, Md., 1987, p. 9.
18. Ibid., p. 8.
19. National Center for Health Statistics. Characteristics of American Indian and Alaska native births, United States, 1984. Prepared by Taffel SM. Monthly Vital Statistics Report, Vol. 36, No. 3 Suppl. DHHS Pub. No. (PHS)87-1120. Hyattsville, Md., 1987.

20. National Center for Health Statistics. Births of Hispanic parentage, 1985. *Op. cit.*
21. National Center for Health Statistics. Advance report of final natality statistics, 1985. *Op. cit.*, table 2, p. 14.
22. National Center for Health Statistics. Prenatal care, United States, 1969–75. Prepared by Taffel SM. Vital and Health Statistics, Series 21, No. 33. DHEW Pub. No. (PHS)78-1911. Washington, D.C.: Government Printing Office, 1978.
23. Singh S, Torres A, and Forrest JD. The need for prenatal care in the United States: Evidence from the 1980 National Natality Survey. Fam. Plan. Perspect. 17:118–124, 1985.
24. National Center for Health Statistics. Advance report of final natality statistics, 1985. *Op. cit.*, p. 7.
25. National Center for Health Statistics. Births of Hispanic parentage, 1985. *Op. cit.*, p. 9.
26. Singh S et al. *Op. cit.*, p. 121.
27. Ventura SJ and Hendershot GE. Infant health consequences of childbearing by teenagers and older mothers. Public Health Rep. 99:138–146, 1984, p. 144.
28. Placek P. The 1980 National Natality Survey and National Fetal Mortality Survey: Methods used and PHS agency participation. Public Health Rep. 99:111–116, 1984.
29. National Center for Health Statistics. National Survey of Family Growth, Cycle III sample design weighting, and variance estimation. Prepared by Bachrach C, Horn MC, Mosher WD, and Shitmizu I. Vital and Health Statistics, Series 2, No. 98. Washington, D.C.: Government Printing Office, 1985.
30. Singh S et al. *Op. cit.*
31. Unpublished data from the 1982 National Survey of Family Growth, provided by the Family Growth Statistics Branch, Division of Vital Statistics, National Center for Health Statistics, U.S. Public Health Service.
32. Johnson S et al. *Op. cit.*, p. 19.
33. Singh S et al. *Op. cit.*, p. 120.
34. *Ibid.*, p. 123.
35. Ingram DD, Makuc D, and Kleinman JC. National and state trends in use of prenatal care, 1970–83. Am. J. Public Health 76:415–423, 1986, p. 417.
36. Hughes D et al. *Op. cit.*, p. 70.
37. Kalmuss D et al. *Op. cit.*, p. ii.
38. Ingram DD et al. *Op. cit.*
39. Johnson K, Rosenbaum S, and Simons J. The Data Book. Washington, D.C.: Children's Defense Fund, 1985.
40. Hughes D, Johnson K, Rosenbaum S, and Simons J. Maternal and Child Health Data Book: The Health of America's Children. Washington, D.C.: Children's Defense Fund, 1986.
41. Hughes D, Johnson K, Rosenbaum S, Simons J, and Butler E. The Health of America's Children: Maternal and Child Health Data Book. Washington, D.C.: Children's Defense Fund, 1987.
42. Hughes D et al. The Health of America's Children: Maternal and Child Health Data Book. 1988. *Op. cit.*
43. National Center for Health Statistics. Prenatal care, United States, 1969–75. *Op. cit.*
44. Ingram DD et al. *Op. cit.*, p. 420.
45. *Ibid.*, p. 421–422.
46. *Ibid.*, p. 415.
47. Johnson K. The demographics of prenatal care utilization. Paper prepared for the Committee on Outreach for Prenatal Care. Institute of Medicine, Washington, D.C., 1988.

Barriers to the Use of Prenatal Care

Interventions to increase the use of prenatal care should be based on a firm understanding of why some pregnant women do not obtain adequate prenatal supervision. As a step in that direction, this chapter outlines a variety of barriers to care that many women face. Four categories of obstacles are discussed:

1. a set of financial barriers ranging from problems in private insurance and Medicaid to the complete absence of health insurance;
2. inadequate capacity in the prenatal care system relied on by low-income women;
3. problems in the organization, practices, and atmosphere of prenatal services themselves; and
4. cultural and personal factors that can limit use of care.

FINANCIAL BARRIERS

The average bill for having a baby is about $4,300—a figure that includes hospital and physician charges spanning prenatal care, labor and delivery services, a postpartum checkup, and hospital services for the newborn.[*][1] Considering that the typical annual income of a couple in their

---

*This figure includes both complicated and uncomplicated pregnancies and deliveries as well as costs associated with health problems in some newborns.

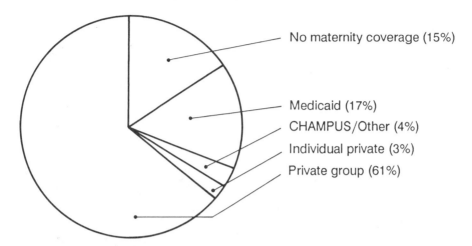

FIGURE 2.1   Percentage distribution of all new mothers by insurance coverage at time of delivery, United States, 1985. SOURCE: Gold RB, Kenney AS and Singh S. Paying for maternity care in the United States. Fam. Plan. Perspect. 19:190–211, 1987, table 12.

early 20's—the prime childbearing years—is about $19,800,[2] pregnancy and childbirth can be a great financial burden. It is therefore not surprising that financial status, and health insurance coverage in particular, plays a major role in determining whether or not prenatal care is secured. Despite the importance of health insurance, an increasing number of Americans—some 37 million at present—are without any. Even those who do have insurance may have little or no coverage for maternity care.

In this section, three aspects of the insurance problem are discussed: (1) gaps in private insurance coverage for maternity services; (2) the role of Medicaid in helping some, but not all, poor women secure prenatal care; and (3) the problems of women with no health insurance at all. An excellent analysis of these issues has been published by the Alan Guttmacher Institute (AGI).[3] The sections that follow draw heavily on that report.

To provide background and context for these sections, Figure 2.1 shows the type of maternity coverage reported for women who gave birth in 1985. Although these data reflect payment source at time of delivery and not payment source for prenatal care exclusively, the two sources generally correspond quite closely.

Private Insurance

Privately insured women are more likely to obtain adequate prenatal care than uninsured or Medicaid-enrolled women. The reasons for this differential include the demographic characteristics of privately insured women (higher income, more education, and so on), the greater availability of providers to women with private insurance (which, in turn, is related to more generous reimbursement patterns and other factors), and the ability of these women to pay in advance for selected prenatal services.

Some 41 million women (73 percent of women between the ages of 15 and 44) are now covered by private health plans.[4] Most private coverage derives from group insurance, obtained by women on their own or through their spouse or family as an employment benefit. Since the enactment of the Pregnancy Discrimination Act in 1978, employers have been required to offer maternity care benefits in the same manner as other medical benefits. As a result, many more private plans now include maternity coverage. In 1977, only 57 percent of employees with new health insurance policies had maternity care benefits, but by 1982 the number had increased to 89 percent.[5]

Many women do not have access to employer-based group coverage because they or their spouses are unemployed or work for employers who do not offer health benefits. Moreover, if the cost to the employee is too high, the mere availability of an employer-based group insurance plan does not ensure enrollment. In fact, even enrollment does not guarantee that a woman will be adequately covered for maternity care or protected from high cost-sharing burdens. Gaps in coverage, imposition of waiting periods that may exclude women already pregnant, recent cutbacks in dependent coverage under some plans, the growing reluctance of employers to help finance dependent coverage, shifts and increases in premiums, and deductible and copayment requirements have all placed new and complex burdens on women and young families. A few of these problems in private insurance are discussed in more detail below.

Eligibility for Coverage Although over 80 percent of all privately insured Americans under age 65 are insured through their employers, over half of uninsured individuals in 1985 were in families where at least one member had a full-time job.[6] Whether employers furnish insurance depends on their financial status, on how highly they choose to compensate their work force, or both. Small businesses and employers of low-paid or part-time nonmanufacturing and seasonal workers are less likely to furnish health insurance or to underwrite the cost of premiums.[7] Since women are disproportionately represented in these categories of workers, they are less likely to be insured.[8] Firms that pay low wages are substantially less likely to offer subsidized health insurance as part of their employees benefit packages, even though it is lower paid employees who are particularly in need of the subsidy.[9] Moreover, in recent years employers who do subsidize employee coverage have begun to reduce or in some instances eliminate their contributions.[10] This trend has particularly serious implications for women employed at minimum wage jobs, since the minimum wage has remained fixed and unadjusted for inflation since 1980.

Women who are not in the labor force are almost entirely dependent for private insurance on their spouses' family coverage through employers' plans. Thus, women who are not married and are unemployed or marginally employed are significantly more likely than women who are married or employed full-time to have no private insurance. Similarly, nonworking women in poor and near-poor families are particularly likely to be without private insurance because their spouses, like low-income workers generally, tend to have no employer-based insurance, to have employer-based insurance covering the working spouse only, or to have access only to coverage that is too costly to buy. The increase in single-parent families (whether headed by a divorced or separated parent or a never-married parent) has also contributed to the growing number of families without private coverage. Single-parent families are three to four times more likely to be completely uninsured than two-parent families.[11]

Even women who have coverage may face long waiting periods before benefits can be obtained. The AGI report notes that:

... 58 percent of full-time employees participating in employment related health insurance programs—including about 20 million women of reproductive age—belong to plans that require a waiting period ... 18 percent [of such employees] belong to plans that impose waiting periods of 10 months or more, thus effectively precluding any reimbursement for care during pregnancy.[12]

Scope and Depth of Coverage   Employees and families with private insurance are increasingly likely to be covered less comprehensively than they were in the past. The Pregnancy Discrimination Act of 1978, which mandates that private insurance plans provide coverage of routine maternity care, does not apply to employers of fewer than 15 persons, and not all states have enacted remedial legislation of their own to close this gap. Furthermore, such state laws, where applicable, do not apply to employers who self-fund their insurance coverage. As a result, some five million women have insurance plans with virtually no coverage for maternity care.[13]

In addition, insurers have varying policies regarding coverage of laboratory, X-ray, and other supplemental services such as nutritional counseling. Some private insurance plans either fail to cover benefits that may be important to pregnancy outcomes or impose limits on coverage unrelated to medical need. For example, in 1985 only 55 percent of private plans covered home health care.[14]

Patient Cost-Sharing Except for prepaid health plans, first-dollar coverage of prenatal and delivery costs is seldom included in private health insurance packages. Pregnant women usually pay an initial deductible, and physicians generally require a relatively large payment in advance for prenatal care. At the time of delivery, pregnant women may also be asked to pay a percentage of hospital room charges (typically 20 percent, sometimes more). Recent employer cost-containment strategies have included significant increases in deductibles and coinsurance obligations, which pass the cost directly on to the individual. Although adequate data on out-of-pocket costs for pregnancy and childbirth among privately insured women are unavailable, it is apparent that, for some women, the required cash payments are significant and burdensome.

Medicaid

The Medicaid program is the largest single source of health care financing for the poor and is generally believed to be primarily responsible for the increased use of medical services by low-income individuals since its enactment in 1965. With regard to prenatal care specifically, the National Center for Health Statistics' (NCHS) natality data from 1969 (the first year in which NCHS compiled such data) and 1980 show significant improvements in the use of prenatal care shortly after Medicaid was enacted and 11 years later, as evidenced by increases in the proportion of pregnant women seeking care in the first trimester (Table 1.11). Since 1980 there has been little improvement, as discussed in Chapter 1. Table 1.11 shows that the greatest increase in use of prenatal care between 1969 and 1980 was among black women. In 1969, 43 percent of black women and 72 percent of white women initiated prenatal care in the first trimester of pregnancy. These figures increased to 63 percent for black women and 79 percent for white women in 1980. These differential gains may be due to the fact that higher proportions of black women were living in poverty and enrolled in Aid to Families with Dependent Children (AFDC—that is, welfare) during this period, and AFDC enrollment has traditionally included eligibility for Medicaid benefits. These findings underscore the special role of Medicaid in increasing minority access to prenatal care.

Selected state reports confirm the importance of Medicaid in securing prenatal services. For example, Norris and Williams examined the impact of Medi-Cal (California's Medicaid program) on perinatal outcomes in California and found major differentials in prenatal care use among selected ethnic groups between 1968 and 1978, a period of significant Medi-Cal expansion. In 1968, Medi-Cal reimbursed costs for 13 percent of all California births; in 1978, it reimbursed 27 percent. Although the proportion of women receiving care in the first trimester increased for all groups in the state during that period (whether enrolled in Medi-Cal or not), the increase was greatest among enrolled women. For example, among white (non-Spanish surname) women on Medi-Cal, 46 percent began prenatal care during the first trimester in 1968; by 1978, that figure had grown to 65 percent—a gain of almost 20 percentage points. Among white (non-Spanish surname) women not enrolled in Medi-Cal, the improvement was more modest: 76 percent began care in the first trimester in 1968 versus 82 percent in 1978.[15]

Despite such favorable trends, data also show that women covered by Medicaid do not obtain prenatal care as early in pregnancy or make as many visits to providers as women with private insurance. For example, using data from New York City in 1981, Cooney compared delayed care among Medicaid recipients with delayed care among women with less than 12 years' education (a proxy measure for low income) who had private insurance. In 23 out of 30 subgroups defined by race, marital status, and age, more Medicaid recipients obtained delayed care than women with third-party insurance.[16] Similarly, a 1986 survey of over 2,000 women in Texas found that 85 percent of women with private health insurance began prenatal care in the first trimester versus 40 percent of women enrolled in Medicaid; about 5 percent of privately insured women had five or fewer prenatal visits versus 25 percent of women in Medicaid.[17] Data from the National Survey of Family Growth and several other state surveys confirm this general picture.[18,19]

It is important to add, however, that few of these studies analyzing use of prenatal care by insurance coverage control for the changing eligibility status of women over the course of a pregnancy. In particular, a woman listed as Medicaid-enrolled at the time of delivery may not have become eligible for the program until just before delivery. If, in addition, she delayed beginning prenatal care, she will be counted as a Medicaid-enrolled woman who began care late, even though her delay in beginning care and her Medicaid status may or may not have been related.

Despite this methodological problem, at least three factors suggest that these studies are accurate in their finding that Medicaid is associated with more limited prenatal care than is private insurance. First, as discussed later in this chapter, the Medicaid enrollment process is so time-consuming that a woman may be well into her pregnancy before her eligibility is established. Thus, she may have been financially unable to obtain care earlier. Second, Medicaid-insured women rely more heavily on clinics for prenatal care than do women with private insurance, and in many communities these clinics are overburdened and unable to schedule appointments promptly.[20] Also, the number of physicians accepting Medicaid-enrolled pregnant women has always been limited and in some areas it is decreasing. (These issues of system capacity are taken up later in

TABLE 2.1   Annual Visits to the Doctor and Other Characteristics of
Poor Women[a] with an Infant Age 3 Months or Younger, National
Health Interview Survey, 1978, 1980, and 1982

	Poor Women		
Characteristic	Uninsured (N = 71)	Medicaid (N = 98)	Other Insurance (N = 132)
Annual visits to doctor (no.)	11.0	12.6	13.1
Black (%)	19.7	42.9	18.2
Community type (%)			
Central city	28.2	48.0	28.0
Rural	56.3	19.4	40.2
Region (%)			
Northeast	9.9	23.5	17.5
South	53.5	24.5	43.9
North central	15.5	31.6	25.0
West	21.1	20.4	13.6
Education (years)	10.9	10.6	11.7
Family income ($ 1982)	1,672	1,438	2,429
Marital status and age (%)			
Unmarried, 17–19	9.9	21.4	3.8
Unmarried, 20+	8.5	45.9	6.1
Married, 17–19	12.7	5.1	12.1
Fair or poor health (%)	14.1	17.3	12.1

NOTE: Insurance status reflects coverage at some time during the interview year. It
was not possible to identify when during the pregnancy coverage of a given type began.
Also, this sample included poor women with an infant age 3 months or younger at the time
of the interview. Their reported annual visits to a doctor largely reflect prenatal care;
however, a postpartum visit and visits not directly related to the pregnancy were also
included in each woman's total count of visits.

[a]Real income per family member of less than $3,500 in 1982 dollars.

SOURCE: 1978, 1980, 1982 National Health Interview Surveys; calculations by J.
Hadley for the Office of Technology Assessment, U.S. Congress.

this chapter.) Finally, women on Medicaid are, by definition, at the bottom
rung of the economic ladder and are characterized by numerous other
demographic factors associated with insufficient prenatal care, including
having limited education, being unmarried, under 20, and in fair or poor
health. (See Table 2.1, although note that the table only reports on poor
women; if Medicaid-enrolled women were compared with all women,
evidence of their disadvantage would be more striking.) Given these
attributes of the Medicaid population, health insurance alone is unlikely to
close the gap between their use of health services and that of more affluent
women with private coverage.

It is not as clear how Medicaid-enrolled women compare with uninsured women in their use of prenatal care. Some studies find that uninsured women receive quantitatively more adequate care than Medicaid-enrolled women. For example, a 1986 survey of 517 births in Rhode Island found that 84 percent of women with private insurance, 70 percent of uninsured women, and 57 percent of Medicaid-insured women obtained adequate prenatal care.[21] By contrast, a General Accounting Office (GAO) study of 1,157 pregnancies found that both Medicaid-enrolled and privately insured women began care earlier in pregnancy and saw a provider more frequently than did women with no insurance.[22] Hadley examined the use of prenatal care by pooling data from the 1978, 1980, and 1982 Health Interview Surveys. He found that when analysis is confined to poor women only—that is, when poverty is held constant—Medicaid-enrolled women made more visits to a doctor than uninsured women, though less than privately insured women (Table 2.1).

The picture that emerges from these many data sets is that Medicaid has improved access to prenatal care for poor women. Enrolled women, however, still do not obtain as much prenatal care as women with private insurance, whether measured by trimester in which care was begun or number of visits. On the other hand, enrolled women probably obtain more prenatal care than uninsured women (when poverty is held constant), although the data on this relationship are mixed.

Despite the importance of Medicaid in helping many low-income individuals (including pregnant women) gain access to health care, a substantial proportion of the poor is not covered by this program. In fact, in 1988 the average income eligibility ceiling for Medicaid was only 49 percent of the federal poverty level.[23] Though designed to meet the medical needs of the disadvantaged, Medicaid in 1985 "reached less than half the people under the federal poverty level in 36 states and in 22 of those states it reached less than a third."[24] In addition, the proportion of the poor covered by Medicaid has decreased: it is estimated that in 1976, 65 percent of the poor were covered by Medicaid; in 1984, the comparable figure is 38 percent.[25]

Aware of the inadequate coverage of Medicaid for many pregnant women and children, Congress has recently expanded eligibility for Medicaid by means of the Deficit Reduction Act of 1984, the Consolidated Ominibus Budget Reconciliation Act of 1985, the Omnibus Budget Reconciliation Acts of 1986 and 1987, and the Medicare Catastrophic Coverage Act of 1988. Two of the most important reforms in these laws are (1) removing the consideration of "household composition" from eligibility determinations for pregnant women and (2) severing the link between Medicaid and AFDC. The 1986 law allowed states for the first time to offer Medicaid to poor children (up to age 5) and to pregnant women with incomes up to 100 percent of the federal poverty level, regardless of their eligibility for welfare or cash assistance under a state's AFDC guidelines. Two-thirds of the states chose to adopt this expansion, and the 1988 law requires all states to have such coverage by 1990. The 1987 law permits states to expand eligibility even further for poor children (up to age 1) and for pregnant women with incomes up to 185 percent of the federal poverty level. As of June 1988, six states had done so.[26] The importance of separating Medicaid from welfare merits emphasis. It affords states the opportunity to increase Medicaid eligibility for particular subgroups, and to receive federal matching funds, without increasing AFDC program costs.

Also available to states are two other important means of severing health care financing from welfare in certain ways and for certain groups: "medically needy" programs and coverage of two-parent families with an unemployed parent (so-called AFDC-UP or Medicaid-UP programs). These option and the newer ones noted above are described by the American Hospital Association in *Medicaid Options: State Opportunities and Strategies for Expanding Eligibility*.[27]

Congress is considering additional reforms to increase Medicaid enrollment among eligible pregnant women and children. For example, a recent legislative proposal would expand Medicaid to help finance casefinding and other activities to identify eligible individuals and assist them in enrolling in the program. The legislation would also require states to maintain an adequate number of obstetrical providers in the program.

Uninsured Women

Despite economic recovery and rising employment, lack of health insurance has become an increasingly important social and economic problem in the United States in recent years. By the mid-1980s, more than 37 million Americans were completely uninsured.

Women of childbearing age are disproportionately represented among the uninsured.[28] An estimated 26 percent of women of reproductive age (14.6 million) have no insurance to cover maternity care, and two-thirds of these (9.5 million) have no insurance at all.

Of poor women, 35 percent are completely uninsured. As one might anticipate, the women that are most likely to be uninsured are the most likely to be poor—those who are black or Hispanic, poorly educated, working in low-paying jobs or unemployed, unmarried, or in their early 20's.[29]

Poor women with no insurance face significant obstacles to obtaining prenatal care. Their options are limited to charity care at the hands of willing providers or care in public health clinics and other settings usually financed by public funds. As the section on system capacity below notes, in many areas these clinics are so overburdened that prompt entry into care can be very difficult.

Provision of free care in clinics and other settings can soften the effects of being uninsured. For example, the GAO study referred to earlier reported that:

> . . . about 86 percent of the interviewees at Cooper Green Hospital in Birmingham, Alabama, where free prenatal care is available through the public health department, were uninsured mothers. Yet, none of these women who received insufficient care cited lack of money as their most important barrier. By contrast, about 27 percent of the women delivering at Los Angeles County–USC Medical Center who obtained insufficient care cited lack of money as the most important barrier. About 94 percent of the births at the hospital were to uninsured mothers. Los Angeles County clinics charge $20 per visit for the first seven prenatal care visits.[30]

It is not known how extensive the availability of free care is nationally or what recent trends have been, although a recent survey suggests that state maternal and child health agencies are able to finance only a small portion of the prenatal care needed by uninsured women—those most likely to seek free or reduced cost care.[30a]

Unfortunately, the proportion of women age 15 to 44 who have no health insurance is likely to grow. Women increasingly work in industries least likely to offer health insurance (such as service and retail jobs); they are also increasingly likely to work part-time, which usually carries no health insurance benefits.[31] Other reasons were noted earlier: growing gaps in the employer-based insurance system and the decreasing proportion of the poor covered by Medicaid. Although expansions of Medicaid will help finance care for some portion of uninsured women, the problem of absent health insurance has outstripped the remedial steps taken thus far.

To sum up, three major themes emerge from the extensive data on the relationship between use of prenatal care and the availability of private insurance, Medicaid, or no insurance. First, women with private insurance are more likely to obtain sufficient prenatal care than those with Medicaid coverage or no insurance, although there are troubling gaps in private insurance coverage. Second, Medicaid has undoubtedly increased access to prenatal care for low-income individuals, but many poor women are not covered by the program, particularly in the first months of pregnancy. Third, a significant number of women have no insurance at all and must depend on charity care, publicly financed clinics, or other resources to obtain prenatal services. The size of this last group is likely to expand.

INADEQUATE SYSTEM CAPACITY

Inadequate capacity in the maternity care system often used by low-income women constitutes a second barrier to use of prenatal care. This section outlines two closely related aspects of the capacity issue: first, inadequate numbers of, and long waiting times for appointments at, facilities such as Community Health Centers and health department clinics—settings that have traditionally provided prenatal care to those unable or unwilling to use the private care system; and second, problems concerning the availability of maternity care providers including the uneven distribution of physicians nationally, the unwillingness of some physicians to care for Medicaid-enrolled pregnant women, and the mal-practice problem.

Services in Organized Settings

Women with limited financial resources, especially women with neither public nor private health insurance, frequently seek prenatal care in so-called "organized settings," as distinct from private physicians in office-based practices. These settings include hospital outpatient depart-ments, Community Health Centers and Migrant Health Centers, public health departments, Maternity and Infant Care projects, and school-based prenatal services.

Several national surveys confirm that these settings are important sources of care for poor women and for young, unmarried, black, or Hispanic women—the same groups at risk for inadequate use of prenatal care. For example, the 1982 National Survey of Family Growth (NSFG) revealed that, although private doctors are the major source of care for both poor and nonpoor women (54 and 83 percent, respectively), clinics are much more important for poor women (that is, women with incomes of less than 150 percent of the federal poverty level). About 39 percent of poor women used clinics, compared to 12 percent of nonpoor women. The NSFG also showed that, among pregnant women, about 36 percent of Hispanic women, 45 percent of black women, 42 percent of women under age 20, and 47 percent of unmarried women went to a clinic for their first prenatal visit, as compared with about 10 to 15 percent of white, older, and married women.[32] Women enrolled in Medicaid were particularly inclined to seek prenatal care at clinics: 60 percent of women whose delivery was paid for at least in part by Medicaid obtained prenatal care at a clinic versus 21 percent of all women.[33] The 1980 National Medical Care Utilization and Expenditures Survey (NMCUES) also shows that poor, minority, and single pregnant women rely heavily on clinics for prenatal care.[34]

The special value of these clinics—these organized settings—stems from at least three factors. First, as just noted, they typically provide prenatal care to uninsured or Medicaid-enrolled women. Second, the poor, the very young, and persons not part of mainstream culture often need intensive health education and require assistance in areas beyond medical care, such as housing, welfare, and nutrition. Organized settings are usually able to link women to a broader array of services than office-based private physicians are, and clinics often provide more comprehensive care, including, for example, classes in preparation for childbirth and parenting. Finally, some data indicate that pregnant women in these settings begin prenatal care earlier and receive more visits than comparable groups of pregnant women using other systems of care.[35]

Several data sources suggest that there is a growing demand for prenatal services in clinics—a picture consistent with the increasing number of women of reproductive age without adequate private health insurance and the decreasing number of private providers caring for Medicaid-enrolled and other low-income women (see below). The Public Health Foundation, for example, reports that reliance on public health clinics for prenatal care has been increasing. State Health Agencies provided clinical services to 12 percent of pregnant women in fiscal year (FY) 1981, 13 percent in FY 1983, and nearly 15 percent in FY 1985. The percentage of women receiving prenatal care in local public health agencies is probably higher because of underreporting to the state department of health.[36]

Community Health Centers (CHCs) and Migrant Health Centers (MHCs) have also emerged as major sources of care for poor families. Some 5.5 million persons obtain health care through these centers and prenatal services are an important part of the comprehensive services provided. The Bureau of Health Care Delivery and Assistance estimates that in 1986 the CHC–MHC network provided prenatal care to more than 118,000 women. The demand for perinatal services (both prenatal and delivery care) through these clinics has increased steadily during the 1980s.[37]

Hospital clinics are another important source of prenatal services, especially for women with high-risk pregnancies. In some urban neighborhoods, hospital clinics are virtually the only source. Although national data on the number of such hospital services and on trends in patient load are unavailable, numerous anecdotes suggest that in some communities demand for care in these clinics has increased dramatically in recent years.

Are there enough of these clinics and enough appointment slots in each to care promptly for the women who seek services in these settings? Reports from several sources suggest that the answer is no. For example:

a. Brooks and Miller compared information obtained in 1978–1979 and in 1982–1983 from 15 local health departments geographically dispersed throughout the United States. In part because of reduced federal funding and a deep recession in the 4 years between studies, the departments as a group had smaller budgets and staffs, experienced a greater demand for their services, and were forced to accentuate income-producing services.

Most of the 15 reported reduction or elimination of maternity services, nutrition services, or both.[38]

b. In September 1985, the Los Angeles County Department of Health Services surveyed its 42 public health clinics and comprehensive health centers offering prenatal care. Twenty-five of these clinics had waiting times of more than 2 weeks for an initial prenatal appointment; the median waiting time in these 25 clinics was 21 days, and 16 had waiting times ranging from 4 to 14 weeks.[39] As one of the authors of this backlog study said, "A woman has to call for an appointment before she gets pregnant to get an appointment before the end of her first trimester."[40]

c. In a national survey of barriers to prenatal care, the General Accounting Office cited numerous instances of limited capacity. For example, "according to the nurse coordinator at the Charleston [West Virginia] prenatal care clinic, the clinic has had to close admissions once a year for the past 4 years because of high patient volume and limited staff. Clinic personnel in mid-November 1986 . . . said that they would accept no new patients until mid-January, 1987."[41]

d. In a recent 3-month period (June through August 1986) in San Diego County, 1,245 women seeking prenatal care were turned away by publicly financed community clinics because the clinics were filled to capacity. Similarly, in Orange County, California, 2,000 women who turned to the county's prenatal clinics in 1985 could not get appointments. County health officials estimated that half of the patients who could not be cared for at county clinics were unable to obtain prenatal care elsewhere in the county.[42]

e. A survey in 1982 of 12 private, nonprofit hospitals in New York City revealed waiting times for a first prenatal appointment of up to four months.[43]

In the absence of comprehensive state or national data, it is impossible to determine how widespread such system overload is or whether other care networks have been able to meet changing needs. Numerous reports suggest, however, that in some communities the capacity of the clinic systems relied on by low-income women is so limited that prompt care is not always available and that in some additional areas care is unavailable altogether. It is important to stress that adequate, even excess, capacity can exist for affluent women in the same geographic area as inadequate capacity for low-income women.

Maternity Care Providers

Capacity also hinges on the distribution and practice patterns of providers. Obviously, maldistribution of physicians can affect a woman's ability to secure adequate, timely prenatal care. While there are more physicians per capita in the United States than in virtually any other country, some communities do not have enough physicians to meet their needs and others have no physicians at all. In New York State, for example, there are 220 physicians per 100,000 persons, compared with only 80 per 100,000 in Mississippi; the national average is 140 per 100,000. More than 5,000 communities, most of them rural, have no doctor.[44]

The uneven distribution of providers is a particularly serious problem in maternity care. In 1983, the state of Mississippi reported to the President's Commission on Ethical Problems in Medicine that 51 of its 82 counties had no obstetrician.[45] Similarly, 11 of California's 58 counties have no board-certified obstetrician–gynecologist, and 9 of these counties have no public prenatal care clinic either.[46] The American College of Obstetricians and Gynecologists reports that, although the number of residents and practicing obstetricians per 100,000 persons has been increasing, one-fourth of 577 areas in the United States (defined by zip codes) have fewer than four obstetricians per 100,000, and 38 of the 577 areas have no obstetrician at all.[47]

Even in communities with an adequate supply of providers, poor and uninsured pregnant women may not have access to care unless providers are willing to accept their form of payment. Large numbers of obstetricians in particular do not accept Medicaid as payment, and many more will not take patients who are uninsured. For example, a 1985 California survey found that 15 of the state's 58 counties had no obstetrician who would accept Medi-Cal patients—even though more than 13,000 women of childbearing age who were eligible for Medi-Cal lived in those counties.[48] Among primary care physicians, obstetricians have been tagged as the least likely to accept Medicaid patients. Mitchell and Schurmann reported that between 1977 and 1980, nearly 36 percent of all obstetricians said they did not provide care to Medicaid patients, compared with 25 percent of general practitioners, 23 percent of pediatricians, and 20 percent of physicians in internal medicine.[49] A 1983 national survey of private physicians who provide obstetric care found that 44 percent did not accept Medicaid reimbursement.[50] Moreover, there is evidence that overall provider participation in Medicaid (including providers of obstetric care) has decreased in recent years.[51]

Several reasons have been cited for the limited and declining participation in Medicaid of obstetricians and other maternity care providers: inefficient processing of Medicaid claims and burdensome paper work leading to delays in reimbursement; payment through a global fee rather than a per-visit fee; and a feeling that the risk of malpractice claims in a Medicaid population is greater than in other populations. The most important deterrents, however, appear to be rising malpractice costs (discussed below) and reimbursement rates that represent only a fraction of cost or of privately reimbursed fees.

With regard to reimbursement, the Alan Guttmacher Institute found in 1986 that physicians' usual charges averaged $830 for a vaginal delivery and $1,040 for a cesarean section; both figures included prenatal care. Medicaid reimbursement for these services was substantially lower. For example, although the maximum reimbursement for a normal vaginal delivery averaged $554, the range among states was substantial—from $216 in New Hampshire to $1,027 in Massachusetts.[52] Although Medicaid reimbursement rates have risen in recent years—quite substantially in a few states—they remain below physicians' usual charges.

The problem of low Medicaid reimbursement is exacerbated by the high proportion of Medicaid women who are high-risk patients. Because of multiple health and social problems, these women often need more frequent and comprehensive maternity care than more affluent women, and such extra care can be time-consuming and expensive to provide. Indeed, the case could be made that, because many pregnant women enrolled in Medicaid are at high risk, reimbursement for their care should be greater than average fees.

The availability of nurse–practitioners and certified nurse–midwives (CNMs) deserves special comment in this discussion of system capacity. Despite the evidence that such personnel are particularly effective in managing the care of pregnant women who are at high risk because of social and economic factors—and that CNMs especially serve disproportionate numbers of women who are poor, adolescent, members of minority groups, and residents of inner cities or rural areas—legal restrictions and obstetrical customs limit their numbers and scope of practice.[53] At present, only about 2,600 CNMs are actively in practice in the United States, even though in many European nations they provide the majority of maternity services.

Malpractice

Underlying this complicated issue of a limited pool of providers is the current malpractice situation. In recent years, obstetrical providers' medical malpractice insurance costs have risen dramatically—doubling between 1982 and 1985—because of changes in medical technology, the use of national rather than local standards of care in assessing malpractice, questions of inadequate supervision and sanction of substandard physicians, large awards in malpractice suits, contingency fees for attorneys, certain insurance company practices, and other factors. These issues and others related to malpractice are discussed in more detail in the paper by Rosenbaum and Hughes, which appears at the end of this volume.

The increase in malpractice insurance premiums and a growing concern about the risk of malpractice litigation are associated with the increasing number of providers who have discontinued or significantly reduced their obstetrical practice. A comparison of 1983 and 1987 surveys of obstetrician–gynecologists reveals that the percentage of respondents indicating decreases in their level of high-risk obstetrical care due specifically to malpractice concerns increased from 18 percent to 27 percent. Malpractice concerns were also linked to a decrease in the number of deliveries that respondents performed and to an increase in the percentage who stopped practicing obstetrics altogether.[54,55] Similarly, in 1986 the American Academy of Family Physicians reported that 23 percent of its members had stopped practicing obstetrics due to malpractice concerns.[56]

Reports from individual states mirror these national trends.[57] For example, an Oregon survey of physicians providing obstetrical services concluded in 1987 that "the availability of obstetrical care in Oregon has become a critical issue over the past few years as increasing numbers of physicians eschew the practice of obstetrics in light of increasing malpractice insurance premiums and a rising probability of litigation."[58] Between 1984 and 1987, 25 percent of the pool of delivery physicians was lost in that state.[59] Community Health Center directors in Florida, Texas, California, and New York report that local obstetricians who used to take referrals from CHCs no longer do so because they have given up obstetrical practice, largely in response to rising insurance costs and concerns about malpractice litigation.[60] In some U.S. communities, particularly those with poorer populations and no teaching or public facilities, obstetrical care may be disappearing entirely.

A closely related effect of the malpractice situation is that publicly financed clinics and health centers are finding it more difficult to obtain liability insurance and to find providers willing to serve in the clinics, thus contributing further to the reduced availability of subsidized maternity care for poor and uninsured women. Such chronically underfunded facilities as inner-city health centers often cannot afford increasingly costly insurance and must therefore cut back on their obstetric services. CHCs' insurance rates have risen so sharply that some centers have been forced to discontinue obstetric care entirely. Policies that cost between $800 and $900 in 1985 cost $12,000 in 1986.[61] Various communities, such as the District of Columbia, report that maintaining prenatal services in public clinics is becoming increasingly difficult because of liability costs and concerns.[62] Confirming these scattered reports, 85 percent of agencies responding to a national survey on reasons for poor provider participation in public programs serving low-income women said that "physicians 'often' say they do not participate because public program fees are insufficient to cover their malpractice [insurance] costs."[63]

ORGANIZATION, PRACTICES, AND ATMOSPHERE OF PRENATAL SERVICES

Although the insurance and capacity problems described in the preceding sections are common barriers to prenatal care, use can also be limited by the way services are organized and provided at the local level. Such problems usually cannot be resolved by giving pregnant women insurance or locating a provider. They stem from inadequate coordination among services, problems in securing Medicaid coverage, and such classic access problems as transportation difficulties, inhospitable provider practices, and cultural barriers. Although many of these problems are experienced primarily by low-income women, they are not limited to the poor. Child care problems, for example, or difficulty in taking time off from work for a prenatal visit, can be experienced by women of all incomes.

Links Among Services

Several federal programs furnish prenatal care and related services to low-income women: Medicaid; the Maternal and Child Health (MCH) Services Block Grant; the Special Supplemental Food Program for Women, Infants, and Children (WIC); Community Health Centers; and Migrant and Rural Health Centers. Each is designed to serve a different function: a source of payment (Medicaid), direct services (MCH Block Grant and health centers), and nutritional supplementation and education (WIC). In theory, these programs can furnish many pregnant women with a wide array of maternity services; in fact, however, the programs are not always carefully coordinated at the local level to ensure optimal benefits. Moreover, links among these publicly financed services, private physicians, and such other service systems as welfare and housing are often fragile to nonexistent.

Without doubt, limited funding of these programs has contributed greatly to their inability to ensure full access to comprehensive care. For example, the Southern Regional Task Force on Infant Mortality reported that, although Congress appropriated $457 million for the MCH Block Grant in FY 1986, all 19 states and territories surveyed by the Task Force claimed that Block Grant funds were insufficient to meet maternity needs.[64] Even when fully funded, however, programs are difficult to coordinate because they are often independent of one another and have separate administering agencies, rules and guidelines, and organizational and political constraints. For example, although a woman may be eligible for both Medicaid and services through a health department clinic, enrolling in both systems may require applying at different sites, meeting different eligibility standards, completing different applications, and furnishing different documentation. Moreover, the programs may rely on different providers. In some states, public health clinics and CHCs are not certified as Medicaid providers, thereby limiting the choices available to pregnant women enrolled in Medicaid.

Similarly, WIC services and prenatal care are not routinely coordinated. A Department of Health and Human Services study showed that, among five sample states where income eligibility for prenatal services and the WIC program were identical, WIC enrollment among the prenatal care patients averaged only 58 percent. Such low rates of participation were attributed to many of the same barriers to coordination that exist between Medicaid and publicly financed prenatal services.[65]

Another important example of poor linkage is the gap between pregnancy testing and prenatal care. Although pregnancy tests are widely available in a variety of settings, anecdotal reports suggest that a positive pregnancy test does not routinely lead to a prompt prenatal care appointment for women who choose to carry the pregnancy to term. Pregnancy-testing sites commonly provide telephone numbers for prenatal services to women receptive to such a referral, but it is less common for a first prenatal visit to be actually scheduled or, if broken, followed up. This gap can be associated with major delays in beginning prenatal care. For example, a study in Hartford, Connecticut, showed that among teenagers under 18 there was a mean delay of almost 5 weeks between confirmation of pregnancy and a first prenatal visit.[66] A study in Ohio found that, among a sample of low-income women, close to 40 percent waited 2 months or more after a positive pregnancy test to contact a prenatal care provider for an appointment.[67] Ambivalence may account for a significant amount of this delay, but the studies also reveal an opportunity for better coordination among systems (see Appendix A).

Whether a woman has a usual source of health care is another aspect of service coordination. Numerous studies have documented greater use of prenatal care among women who regularly use a health care facility than among those who, for example, rely on emergency rooms for episodic care or have no regular health care provider.[68] Such studies suggest that women who have only a marginal connection to the health care system are not likely to establish one during pregnancy.

Medicaid Application Procedures

As described earlier, the Medicaid program is the major source of payment for care obtained by poor pregnant women, yet actual enrollment rates among eligible women are low and vary across states. A study by the National Governor's Association found that state enrollment among women who were newly eligible in the early 1980s ranged from 11 percent to 84 percent. For example, when North Carolina expanded its program to include several new groups of pregnant women, only 1,470 of an estimated 2,100 newly eligible recipients enrolled in the first year. Other states, including Arkansas, Texas, Mississippi, and Florida, report similar shortfalls.[69]

Many problems and complexities in the administration of Medicaid underlie these gaps between potential and actual numbers of program participants. In particular, Medicaid programs rarely invest in publicizing their benefits or how to enroll. Consequently, women may fail to obtain Medicaid coverage because they know little about the program, are unaware of their eligibility, do not know how to apply for coverage, or a combination of all three. For example, a recent survey of state Medicaid programs showed that brochures about the program rarely mention pregnancy as grounds for eligibility, and few conduct any comprehensive activities to let potential recipients know of the program.[70] Given the relentless pressures on Medicaid to contain costs, the disinclination to advertise or to recruit recipients aggressively is not surprising.

Even women who know about Medicaid and try to apply are not assured an easy process, particularly if they are not on welfare already (and thus automatically enrolled in Medicaid) and are eligible for the program only because of their pregnancy. Complicated application forms, a stressful certification procedure, denials of eligibility on the basis of incomplete evidence, requirements of extensive documentation, long delays between application and notification of eligibility, and loss of eligibility during pregnancy are widely reported. Many of these problems can be traced to state and federal regulations shaping the program and to the threat of fines for enrollment errors (in particular, enrolling women who are later found to be ineligible). Investigators from the Alan Guttmacher Institute found, for example, that applications run from 4 to 40 pages long, the average length being 14. They described how intricate the applications can be:

A typical application often includes 80 or 100 questions about the applicant's and her household members' identity, income, assets and outgoings. There are usually questions on the value of any property owned, jewelry, cars, life, health and burial insurance, cash on hand, Christmas fund accounts and many other items of value. Income from numerous sources is counted, including employment, public assistance, interest, scholarships, loans, gifts, free meals received, etc. The education and employment status of each household member is probed as are expenditures for such items as child care, utilities and medical bills. The identity of each household member must be proven by a social security card and/or a birth certificate and virtually every financial item must be documented. A single missing utility bill, apartment lease, rent receipt, or evidence of a checking account balance or child care expenses can cost an individual eligibility for the program. As one would expect, then, it can easily take applicants two or three visits—and sometimes more—to the welfare or social service office to complete the application and supply the required documentation. Each visit can entail a half day at the office, much of it spent waiting to see an eligibility worker, and for some women may entail taking time off work without pay. Moreover, once an individual becomes eligible, any changes in income, expenditures or household composition must be promptly reported under penalty of losing benefits, and eligibility must be redetermined periodically, as required by the state. In most states, a Medicaid card is mailed to recipients monthly to minimize the chances of an ineligible person having use of the card. In the 6 states where Medicaid is administered at the county rather than the state level, additional application forms and procedures may be required.[71]

A lapse of several weeks between application for and notification of eligibility is common. States in the South, for example, report an interval of about 5 weeks. Moreover, if the actual Medicaid card is not sent with the letter notifying a woman she has been found eligible, additional delays in obtaining prenatal care may occur, because some health care providers are reluctant to accept the letter as evidence of enrollment. A recent provision in federal Medicaid law permits states to authorize certain health care providers to make preliminary determinations of Medicaid eligibility for pregnant women and to be reimbursed for providing services to them for 45 days or until eligibility is actually determined—so-called presumptive eligibility. By July 1988, 19 states had adopted a presumptive eligibility program for pregnant women.[72]

Another option open to states that wish to shorten the application process is waiving consideration of assets in determining eligibility. As of June 1988, 25 jurisdictions had completely eliminated use of an assets test, and a few others have simplified and liberalized their means test. States have also recently been given the option of ensuring continuous, uninterrupted coverage for Medicaid-enrolled pregnant women, eliminating the risk of losing coverage in the middle of pregnancy. As of June 1988, 27 jurisdictions had taken advantage of this provision.[73]

The difficult application process, the complexity of the program and the great variations in the program across states create the impression of a system designed to discourage rather than encourage entry into prenatal care. Although Congress and the states have taken a number of steps recently to improve Medicaid—in particular, to broaden eligibility—the program is still limited in its ability to draw low-income women into prenatal care promptly with minimal bureaucratic harrassment.

Classic Barriers to Access

Several classic access barriers, well recognized in the large literature on barriers to health services generally, continue to limit prompt enrollment and continuation in prenatal care. These include problems with transportation and child care, the practices and attitudes of some providers, language barriers, and cultural differences between patients and providers.

Recent work by the GAO and others describes the transportation problems linked to insufficient use of prenatal care—long distances to reach a provider, the high cost of transportation, and no transportation whatever.[74] For example, in Bluefield, West Virginia, many women travel up to 2 hours for prenatal care, and in the Birmingham, Alabama, area, bus transportation is not available in many parts of the county served by the health department.[75] Similarly, the American Nurses' Association describe a county health department that offers prenatal care and that is centrally located to serve an entire region—the county is without public transpor-, tation, however, and women in adjoining counties traveling by bus can get only as far as the county line, which is 15 miles from the clinic.[76]

When prenatal services are not coordinated with public transportation, additional problems can result. Staff at a large Washington, D.C., public hospital report that one reason women fail to keep early morning appointments is that the bus system in the neighborhoods where most patients live does not begin running by the time patients are expected to be at the clinic.[77]

These anecdotes suggest that transportation problems are closely associated with—and may even be seen as a proxy measure of—poverty, particularly the lack of a car and the resulting dependence on imperfect systems of public transportation. In rural areas, where distances to care can be great, the absence of a car can be an insurmountable obstacle.

Medicaid programs are required to cover "medically necessary" transportation costs for enrolled individuals. However, few women know about the option and the process of securing reimbursement is cumbersome.[78] For indigent women not enrolled in Medicaid, little help is avalable to meet transportation costs.

The availability of child care can also affect use of prenatal care. If affordable, convenient child care is difficult to arrange, a pregnant mother may have to bring older children with her to a prenatal care appointment. If there are no child care services nearby or if waiting times for the visit are long, the burden of taking children may outweigh the perceived benefits of the prenatal visit. Studies that ask women about reasons for delayed or no prenatal care confirm that responsibility for other children can interfere with keeping appointments.[79]

Accessibility problems created by long distances to care, inadequate transportation, and lack of child care are compounded by limited clinic hours. Most prenatal services are offered during "normal" working hours (that is, weekdays from, 9:00 a.m. to 5:00 p.m.). For women who work or go to school, the only time available for appointments is usually the lunch hour, when many clinics do not see patients. Even if appointments can be scheduled during the lunch hour, a woman's ability to make such a visit depends on her distance from the provider. If the distance is great—and thus more than an hour is required to complete the visit—women working for hourly wages must forego pay, those in salaried positions risk recrimination for taking too much time off, and those in school miss class time or must miss school altogether. Recently, the District of Columbia began offering prenatal services during evenings and weekends in order to accommodate work and school schedules; it was also recognized that child care is often more easily arranged during evenings and weekends. Patient load increased dramatically at sites with the expanded hours. Although other reforms were also instituted simultaneously, program staff believe that the change in hours was the most important cause of the increased enrollment.[80]

Long clinic waits can be a deterrent to seeking or remaining in prenatal care. In publicly financed clinics, service is often delayed routinely,[81] partly because of block appointments. This system schedules only two groups of appointments a day, one at 8:00 or 9:00 in the morning and another at 1:00 in the afternoon, with patients seen on a first-come, first-served basis. While the first patient who arrives may be seen promptly, the tenth patient may have a 2- or 3-hour wait. Clinics use such systems to make certain that physicians' time is not wasted and to avoid gaps in appointments when patients fail to appear. A wait of several hours can be frustrating and humiliating for the patient, however. Few people have the time—or the patience—to wait long hours, and the costs (in lost wages or school time, extended childcare, and so on) can be burdensome.[82] One study found that low-income women considered the long waiting times at clinics to indicate a disregard for the importance of their time; it was particularly insulting to have only a few minutes with a doctor after waiting several hours for the consultation.[83]

Another practice that influences enrollment in care is that of asking women to wait until at least two menstrual periods have been missed before scheduling a prenatal appointment. Though designed to provide prenatal care only to women whose pregnancies have progressed beyond the first few weeks when miscarriage often occurs, this policy obviously causes delays in onset of care for the majority of pregnant women who do not miscarry.

Use of care can also be influenced by the attitudes and styles of providers, including poor communication about procedures, failure to answer questions, seeing a different provider at each visit, and hurried or otherwise depersonalized care. For example, in a study of determinants of remaining in care in a pediatric setting, Ross and Duff found that when a parent felt the doctor was a good listener, respectful, and willing to give and take, compliance was better than when the physician was seen as insensitive, unwilling to answer questions, and not respectful.[84] Similarly, anecdotal information suggests that clinic "gatekeepers"—such as appointment clerks and receptionists—can discourage continuation in prenatal care by being rude or indifferent. As one woman said, "Getting prenatal care in a clinic is a real hassle, but that's what you have to expect when you're poor."[85]

The difficult relationship and failure of communication between health care providers and low-income clients have been described by many authors.[86] Causes probably include the different socioeconomic and cultural backgrounds of the groups, the awkwardness and stigma often attached to charity care, and cultural differences that affect beliefs about illness and health. Such differences can result in an unfortunate mix of hostility, passivity, and evasiveness on the part of the client, matched by arrogance, testiness, and indifference on the part of the provider.

Language incompatibility exacerbates many barriers. Clinics located in relatively large communities of persons who speak a single, non-English language are likely to have interpreters, if not bilingual providers. However, bilingual providers or medically trained interpreters are not found in most prenatal care settings. Even when children are brought along as interpreters—a very common practice in some areas—communication remains inadequate. An anthropologist describing prenatal clinics for low-income women in New York City noted, "In most of the clinics I visited there was only one interpreter available for every large non-English speaking population. Usually these interpreters were clinic staff members who worked full-time in another capacity. When interpreters were needed they were often not available because they were generally busy with other work."[87]

Experts cite the failure of providers to appreciate the cultural preferences of some patients as an important barrier to care. Among some Hispanic and Asian populations, for example, it is unacceptable to have a pelvic examination done by a man.[88] Yet not all clinics are able to accommodate such preferences, because most physicians are men and not all settings can or will rely on certified nurse–midwives or nurse–practitioners.

The physical surroundings of many prenatal clinics for low-income women—dreary, usually very crowded, and uncomfortable—form another barrier. A study of several New York City prenatal clinics noted that there are usually too few chairs in the waiting rooms, leaving patients to stand in corridors.[89]

Finally, lack of easily available, widely disseminated information about where exactly to go for prenatal services can be an obstacle to care. Studies report that 5 to 18 percent of patients who had obtained little or no care did not know where to seek services.[90–92] Given the relatively poor accessibility of clinic telephone numbers, it is not surprising that this barrier can be significant. Few telephone books, for example, have a listing for "prenatal care" or a similar phrase.

CULTURAL AND PERSONAL BARRIERS

Previous sections have outlined potent barriers to care created by inadequate insurance, limited capacity in the prenatal care system, and the policies and atmosphere of prenatal clinics themselves. It is also apparent that the use of prenatal care is influenced by a woman's attitudes toward her pregnancy and toward prenatal care, her knowledge about such care and whether she sees it as useful, her cultural values and beliefs, a variety of other personal characteristics often called life-style, and certain psychological attributes. This section describes the role of these factors in the use of prenatal care, but it is important to emphasize at the outset that most research on personal barriers does not control for the confounding influence of the prenatal care system itself. That is, little effort has been made to assess the nature and extent of personal barriers to care in different types of prenatal settings.

Attitudes toward pregnancy that may influence efforts to seek prenatal care include whether the pregnancy is planned or unplanned and whether the woman views her pregnancy positively or negatively. Many studies have found that later entry into care and fewer visits are associated with unplanned pregnancy and, similarly, with negative views of a current pregnancy.[93] These attitudes may influence prenatal care in three ways. First, women who did not plan their pregnancy may be less aware of the signs of pregnancy and therefore may recognize their pregnancy later. Second, women who view their pregnancies negatively may delay prenatal care while they decide whether to continue the pregnancy. Finally, an unplanned pregnancy is likely to evoke ambivalent feelings, even in women who decide to continue the pregnancy. This ambivalence may result in late entry into or sporadic use of prenatal care. Here it is important to add that in the United States, more than half of all pregnancies are unplanned.[93a] Given the evidence that unplanned pregnancies are associated with late entry into prenatal care, as noted above, and that the magnitude of unplanned pregnancy in this country is great, it is reasonable to conclude that more extensive use of family planning services would result in reduced rates of late entry into prenatal care.

Attitudes toward prenatal care itself are also influential. Not all women believe that prenatal care is important and worth the effort to seek it out.[94] Some believe that pregnancy is a normal event not needing medical supervision, or that care is needed only if a pregnant woman feels ill; a few women may actually be unaware of what prenatal care is. Previous, unsatisfying experiences with prenatal services may also act as a deterrent. The provider practices and clinic policies outlined above no doubt leave some women with a negative view of prenatal care, reluctant to seek it out in subsequent pregnancies. Studies that have assessed the relationship between attitudes about prenatal care and onset of care show that women who believe the service is important and should be initiated early are more likely to begin care in the first trimester than those attaching less importance to early care.[95,96] The predictive value of positive attitudes toward prenatal care should not be overestimated, however. Oxford et al. noted that, among a sample of women who began care in the third trimester, 42 percent reported that they thought prenatal care should begin during the first few weeks of pregnancy.[97]

Not knowing the signs of pregnancy is also related to use of prenatal services. Studies report that between 16 and 33 percent of women who received insufficient care did not know the signs of pregnancy.[98–101]

Cultural values may affect efforts to seek out prenatal care. Among some cultures, pregnancy is regarded as a healthy condition not requiring medical treatment or a physician's advice.[102] Furthermore, the perception of what constitutes a health problem may vary between patient and provider. In one study, for example, low-income, primarily black women characterized high-risk behavior as not taking prenatal vitamins and catching the flu, but having more than five children or a previous low birthweight infant were not viewed as conditions constituting risk.[103]

Fear as a barrier deserves special comment. There may be at least four types of fear: fear of providers or medical procedures, fear of others' reactions to the pregnancy, fear that one's illegal status in the country will be discovered, and fear that such health-compromising habits as substance abuse or smoking will be uncovered and pressures to change brought to bear. With regard to the first fear, a survey of women who had received no prenatal care found that 52.4 percent indicated fear of hospitals, doctors, or procedures as a primary reason for not seeking care.[104] In her in-depth interviews with disadvantaged women who had suffered an infant death, Boone found that "fear of doctors and nurses represented the single most important factor in their perception of health care providers as inaccessible."[105]

Adolescents are particularly likely to cite fear as a reason for not seeking early care. While some pregnant adolescents fear medical procedures, many also fear the pregnancy itself and parental response. A postpartum teenager who delayed care explained, "When I went to the doctor I was $6\frac{1}{2}$ months—I found out when I was 8 weeks. I didn't go right away because it took me that long to tell my mom."[106] For teenagers who may be eligible for Medicaid during a pregnancy, concerns about confidentiality may be significant. Although procedures vary widely, most states do not have Medicaid policies and practices that protect teenagers' confidentiality. States generally provide a family with only one Medicaid card, which forces teenagers to ask their parents for use of the card before seeking services.[107] Unless they are assured confidentiality, adolescents may choose to protect their secret rather than seek prenatal care.

Another group for whom fear can be a major barrier to prenatal care is illegal immigrants, who may not seek care because they are afraid that they will be reported to the Immigration and Naturalization Service (INS) and eventually deported.[108,109] While reporting is not routine in a clinic, the mere possibility can be a sufficient deterrent. In Los Angeles County, for example, the board of supervisors recently voted to require all persons requesting free or reduced-cost health services to apply first for Medi-Cal, which, in turn, requires completing a form that is sent to the INS. While the policy never went into effect because of a court injunction, it created substantial anxiety among undocumented families. A CHC pediatrician in Los Angeles County reported that the fear generated by the proposal led to an immediate decrease of 50 percent in the number of children attending his clinic.[110]

Pregnant women who are aware that their life-styles place their health and that of their babies at risk may also fear seeking care because they anticipate sanction or pressure to change such habits as drug and alcohol abuse, heavy smoking, and eating disorders. Substance abusers in particular may delay care because of the stress and disorganization that often surround their lives, and because they fear that if their use of drugs is uncovered, they will be arrested and their other children taken into custody.

The issue of drug abuse during pregnancy deserves additional comment. The Chao et al. study in Harlem found that women with insufficient prenatal care were far more likely to report use of heroin, cocaine, or both than women who obtained care early in pregnancy.[111] Poland et al. found that 31 percent of a group of women with inadequate prenatal care abused drugs, mainly heroin, compared with 7 percent of women with more adequate care.[112] Numerous reports detail alarming increases in the proportion of women, including pregnant women, who abuse heroin and cocaine and the resulting rise in the number of babies born with varying degrees of addiction. For example, from January through November 1987, 142 drug-addicted babies were born at a hospital located in a low-income area of Washington, D.C. In 1986, by contrast, there had been 55 such births, and in 1985, 19.[113] Drug abuse among pregnant women has become especially alarming recently because of the hightened risk that these women carry the human immunodeficiency virus (HIV, cause of AIDS), which can be passed on to the developing baby. In some areas of New York City, for example, between 4 and 5 percent of pregnant women are estimated to be infected with the virus.[114]

Homelessness is also associated with poor use of prenatal care. Chavkin et al. compared the use of prenatal services among women living in New York City hotels for the homeless, women living in the city's low-income housing projects, and all other city residents. Forty percent of the hotel residents studied who had given birth between 1982 and 1984 had received no care at all, versus 15 percent of the housing project group and 9 percent of the citywide group. Only 30 percent of the hotel residents had made seven or more visits, versus 58 percent of the housing project group and 68 percent of the citywide group. Unfortunately, homelessness has increased in recent years, and the majority of homeless families are single-parent households headed by women.[115]

Having friends and family to offer emotional support and tangible assistance and having well-developed skills in overcoming isolation, may minimize or eliminate barriers to prenatal care; lack of these assets may constitute an impediment to attaining services. Women vary in the amount of these resources and in their ability to adapt in a stable and organized manner to such major changes in life as pregnancy. Several studies suggest that when emotional support is present—positive interest in the pregnancy by the father, for example, or the presence of someone with whom to share the knowledge of pregnancy—the probability of using prenatal care increases. In the absence of such support, particularly in combination with general social isolation, the likelihood of using prenatal care decreases.[116-118] Similarly, lack of close ties to family and friends may limit use of prenatal care. The importance of these individuals as sources of information about specific clinics or services is well known; if such networks are in disrepair, it will be harder for a woman to connect with needed care.

Stress may decrease a woman's ability to seek prenatal care. For some women, the pressures of daily life are such that prenatal services are of low priority. A study of more than 2,000 women in Massachusetts found that women with inadequate care were significantly more likely than women with adequate care to report being very worried or upset during the pregnancy due to lack of money, problems with the baby's father, housing difficulties, lack of emotional support, and related burdens.[119]

Such factors as depression and, in particular, denial have also been associated with poor use of prenatal care. Although denial that one is pregnant can occur in women of any age, it is often reported in studies of pregnant adolescents. Denial in adolescence often begins as the belief that one is not likely to get pregnant ("It won't happen to me") and continues into pregnancy ("I did not want to accept the fact that I was pregnant").[120,121] Denial is withholding information from oneself; concealment, a related behavior, is the withholding of information from others. Furstenberg reports that one-half of 404 adolescents studied did not tell their parents that they were pregnant for several months. In most cases, the adolescents' mothers either learned of the pregnancy from others or detected it themselves.[122] The prevalence of denial and concealment in adolescents is related to embarrassment about their changing bodies, reluctance to share personal information about their sexuality, lack of knowledge about where to obtain birth control, confusion about the safety and proper practice of contraception, fear of parental disapproval and punishment, and, as noted earlier, fear of pelvic examinations and other medical procedures.[123]

TABLE 2.2   Barriers to the Use of Prenatal Care

I. *Sociodemographic correlates*
Poverty
Inner-city or rural resident
Minority
Under 18 or over 39
Higher parity
Non-English speaking
Unmarried
Less than high school education

II. *System barriers*
Inadequacies in private insurance
policies (waiting periods,
coverage limitations, coinsurance
and deductibles, requirements for
up-front payments)
Absence of either Medicaid or
private insurance coverage of
maternity services
Inadequate or no maternity care
providers for Medicaid-enrolled,
uninsured, and other
low-income women (long wait
to get appointment)
Inadequate transportation services,
long travel time to service sites,
or both
Difficulty obtaining child care
Poor coordination between
pregnancy testing and prenatal
services
Inadequate coordination among
such services as WIC and
prenatal care
Complicated, time-consuming
process to enroll in Medicaid
Availability of Medicaid poorly
advertised
Inconvenient clinic hours,
especially for working women
Long waits to see physician

II. *System barriers* (Continued)
Language and cultural
incompatibility between providers
and clients
Poor communication between clients
and providers, exacerbated by short
interactions with providers
Negative attributes of clinics,
including rude personnel,
uncomfortable surroundings, and
complicated registration procedures
Limited information on exactly
where to get care—phone
numbers and addresses

III. *Barriers based on beliefs, knowledge,*
attitudes, and life-styles
Pregnancy unplanned or viewed
negatively, or both
Ambivalence
Signs of pregnancy not known or
recognized
Prenatal care not valued or
understood
Fear of doctors, hospitals,
procedures
Fear of parental discovery
Fear of deportation or problems
with the Immigration and
Naturalization Service
Fear that certain health habits will
be discovered and criticized
(smoking, eating disorders, drug
or alcohol abuse)
Selected life-styles (drug abuse,
homelessness)
Inadequate social supports and
personal resources
Excessive stress
Denial or apathy
Concealment

Summary

Table 2.2 summarizes the many barriers to use of prenatal care discussed in this chapter, as well as the sociodemographic correlates of prenatal care use defined in Chapter 1. As this daunting list makes clear, many factors that impede use of prenatal care are external to women themselves; they are centered primarily in the financial underpinning of the prenatal care system and in the capacity and practices of various service networks. The pervasive influence of poverty is noteworthy—many of the barriers are strongly associated with low income. The list also helps to show that women's beliefs, knowledge, attitudes, and feelings influence their use of prenatal services, as do such behaviours and conditions as substance abuse and homelessness.

References and Notes

1. Alan Guttmacher Institute. Blessed Events and the Bottom Line: The Financing of Maternity Care in the United States. New York, 1987, p. 18.
2. U.S. Bureau of the Census. Money income of households, families and persons in the United States: 1984. Current Population Reports. Series P-60, No. 151, 1986, table 31.
3. Alan Guttmacher Institute. *Op. cit.* Also published by the Alan Guttmacher Institute as a companion volume is The Financing of Maternity Care in the United States. New York, 1987.
4. Alan Guttmacher Institute. Blessed Events. *Op. cit.*, p. 20.
5. Gold RB and Kenney AM. Paying for maternity care. Fam. Plan. Perspect. 17:103–111, 1985.
6. Chollet D. A Profile of the Non-Elderly Population Without Health Insurance. Washington, D.C.: Employee Benefit Research Institute, 1987.
7. *Ibid.*
8. Gold RB and Kenney AM. *Op. cit.*
9. AS Hansen, Inc. Health Care Survey, January 20, 1986. In Medical Benefits. Charlottesville, Va.: Kelley Communications, 1986, pp. 1–2.
10. Wilensky G, Farley P, and Taylor A. Variations in health insurance coverage: Benefits vs. premiums. Milbank Mem. Fund Q. 62: 134–155, 1984.
11. Sulvetta M and Schwartz C. The Uninsured and Uncompensated Care. Washington, D.C.: National Health Policy Forum, 1986.
12. Alan Guttmacher Institute. Blessed Events. *Op. cit.*, p. 22.
13. *Ibid.*, p. 21.
14. U.S. General Accounting Office. Health Insurance: Comparison of Coverage for Federal and Private Sector Employees. Pub. No. GAO/HRD-87-32BR. Washington, D.C.: Government Printing Office, 1986.
15. Norris FD and Williams RL. Perinatal outcomes among Medicaid recipients in California. Am. J. Public Health 74:1112–1117, 1984.
16. Cooney JP. What determines the start of prenatal care? Medical Care 23:986–997, 1985.
17. Johnson CD and Mayer JP. Texas OB Survey: Determining the Need for Maternity Services in Texas. College Station, Tex.: Public Policy Resources Laboratory, 1987.

18. Pamuk ER, Horn MC, and Pratt WF. Determinants of prenatal care utilization: Data from the 1982 National Survey of Family Growth. Paper presented at the American Public Health Association annual meeting, New Orleans, 1987.
19. See, for example, McDonald TP and Cobrun AF. The Impact of Variations in AFDC and Medicaid Eligibility on Prenatal Care Utilization. Portland: Health Policy Unit, Human Services Development Institute, University of Southern Maine, 1986.
20. Fingerhut LA, Makuc D, and Kleinman JC. Delayed prenatal care and place of first visit: Differences by health insurance and education. Fam. Plan. Perspect. 19:212–214, 1987.
21. O'Connell J. The Association Between Lack of Transportation and Lack of Child Care and the Adequacy of Prenatal Care. Providence: Rhode Island Department of Health, 1987.
22. U.S. General Accounting Office. Prenatal Care: Medicaid Recipients and Uninsured Women Obtain Insufficient Care. Pub. No. GAO/HRD-87-137. Washington, D.C.: Government Printing Office, 1987.
23. Hill I. Reaching Women Who Need Prenatal Care: Strategies for Improving State Perinatal Programs. Washington, D.C.: National Governors' Association, Center for Policy Research, 1988, p. 8.
24. Freedman SA, Klepper BR, Duncan RP, and Bell SP. Coverage of the uninsured and underinsured: A proposal for school enrollment-based family health insurance. N. Engl. J. Med. 18:843–847, 1988, p. 844.
25. Rosenbaum S, Hughes DC, and Johnson D. Maternal and child health services for medically indigent children and pregnant women. Med. Care 26:315–332, 1988, p. 315.
26. Ian Hill, National Governors' Association. Personal communication, 1988.
27. American Hospital Association. Medicaid Options: State Opportunities and Strategies for Expanding Eligibility. Chicago, 1987.
28. National Center for Health Statistics. Health care coverage by sociodemographic and health characteristics, United States. Prepared by Ries P. Vital and Health Statistics, Series 10, No. 162. DHHS Pub. No. (PHS)87-1590. Washington, D.C.: U.S. Public Health Service, 1987.
29. Alan Guttmacher Institute. Blessed Events. Op. cit., p. 43.
30. U.S. General Accounting Office. Op. cit., p. 38.
30a. Rosenbaum S, Hughes DC, and Johnson D. Op. cit.
31. U.S. Bureau of the Census. Statistical Abstract of the United States, 1987. Washington, D.C.: Government Printing Office, 1986, pp. 371–412; and Chollet D. Op. cit., p. 18.
32. Alan Guttmacher Institute. The Financing of Maternity Care. Op. cit., tables 17 and 20.
33. Ibid.
34. Kovar MG and Klerman LV. Who pays for prenatal care? Data from the National Medical Care Expenditure Survey, 1980. Paper delivered at the American Public Health Association annual meeting, Anaheim, California, 1984.
35. Sokol RJ, Woolf RB, Rosen MG, and Weingarden K. Risk, antepartum care and outcome: Impact of a Maternity and Infant Care project. Obstet. Gynecol. 56:150–156, 1980.
36. Public Health Foundation. Unpublished data, 1987.
37. Bureau of Health Care Delivery and Assistance, U.S. Department of Health and Human Services. Unpublished data, 1988.

38. Brooks EF and Miller CA. Recent changes in selected local health departments: Implications for their capacity to guarantee basic medical services. Am. J. Prevent. Med. 3:134–141, 1987.
39. Rogers T, Rhodes K, and Silberman I. Report by the Prenatal Appointment Backlog Task Force. Los Angeles: Programs Division, Department of Health Services, City of Los Angeles Health Department, 1987.
40. Demand for prenatal care bogs down public clinics. Los Angeles Times. November 8, 1987.
41. U.S. General Accounting Office. *Op. cit.*, p. 41.
42. Southern California Child Health Network and the Children's Research Institute of California. Back to Basics: Improving the Health of California's Next Generation. Santa Monica, 1987, pp. 79–80.
43. Kalmuss D, Darabi KF, Lopez I, Caro FG, Marshall E, and Carter A. Barriers to Prenatal Care: An Examination of Use of Prenatal Care Among Low-Income Women in New York City. New York: Community Service Society, 1987.
44. Johnson C. Current Perspectives on Prenatal Care. Lansing, Mich.: University Associates, 1984.
45. President's Commission for the Study of Ethical Problems in Medicine and Biomedical and Behavioral Research. Securing Access to Health Care, Vol. 1. Washington, D.C.: Government Printing Office, 1981, p. 81.
46. Southern California Child Health Network and the Children's Research Institute of California. *Op. cit.*, p. 88.
47. American College of Obstetricians and Gynecologists. Unpublished data, 1987.
48. Dorn S and Dallek G. Medi-Cal Maternity Care and A.B. 3021: Crisis and Opportunity. Los Angeles: National Health Law Program, 1986.
49. Mitchell JB and Schurmann R. Access to private obstetrics/gynecology services under Medicaid. Med. Care 22:1026–1037, 1984.
50. Orr MT and Forrest JD. The availability of reproductive health services from U.S. private physicians. Fam. Plan. Perspect. 17:63–69, 1985.
51. Lewis-Idema D. Provider participation in public programs for pregnant women and children. Washington, D.C.: National Governor's Association, 1988, p. 3.
52. Alan Guttmacher Institute. Blessed Events. *Op. cit.*, p. 34.
53. Committee to Study the Prevention of Low Birthweight. Preventing Low Birthweight. Washington, D.C.: National Academy Press, 1985, pp. 160–161.
54. American College of Obstetricians and Gynecologists. Professional Liability Insurance and Its Effects: Report of a Survey of ACOG's Membership. Washington, D.C., 1983.
55. American College of Obstetricians and Gynecologists. Survey of Professional Liability and Its Effects: Report of a 1987 Survey of ACOG's Membership. Washington, D.C., 1988.
56. American Academy of Family Physicians. Professional Liability Study. Kansas City, Mo., 1986.
57. Lewis-Idema. *Op. cit.*, pp. 21–25.
58. Oregon Medical Association. The Impact of Malpractice Issues on Patient Care: Declining Availability of Obstetrical Services in Oregon. Portland, 1987, p. 1.
59. *Ibid.*, p. 3.
60. See the commissioned paper by Rosenbaum and Hughes at the end of this report.
61. National Association of Community Health Centers. Medical malpractice: Here we go again. Washington, D.C.: NACH newsletter. Winter 1986.

62. Mayor's Advisory Board on Maternal and Infant Health, District of Columbia. Personal communication, 1987.

63. Lewis-Idema. *Op. cit.*, p. 25.

64. Southern Regional Task Force on Infant Mortality, Southern Governors' Association. Unpublished data, 1985.

65. Professional Management Associates, Inc. Improving MCH/WIC Coordination— Final Report and Guide to Good Practices. Report submitted to the Office of the Assistant Secretary of Planning and Evaluation, Department of Health and Human Services. Contract No. HHS-100-84-0069. Washington, D.C., 1986.

66. Christison-Lagay J and Crabtree BF. Barriers Affecting Entry into Prenatal Care: A Study of Adolescents Under 18 in Hartford, Connecticut. Hartford: City of Hartford Health Department, 1984.

67. Toomey BG. Factors Related to Early Entry into Prenatal Care: A Replication. Columbus: Bureau of Maternal and Child Health, Ohio Department of Health, 1985.

68. See, for example, Learner M, Stephens T, Sears JH, and Efirt C. Prenatal Care in South Carolina: Results from the Prenatal Care Survey. Columbia: Department of Health and Environmental Control, 1987. With regard to usual source of care and pediatrics, see Kasper JD. The importance of type of usual source of care for children's physician access and expenditures. Med. Care 25:386–398, 1987.

69. National Governor's Association. Selected State Medicaid Survey. Washington, D.C., 1986.

70. Alan Guttmacher Institute. Blessed Events. *Op. cit.*, p. 32.

71. Alan Guttmacher Institute. The Financing of Maternity Care. *Op. cit.*, pp. 169–170.

72. Ian Hill, National Governors' Association. Personal communication, 1988.

73. *Ibid.*

74. U.S. General Accounting Office. *Op. cit.* See also American College of Obstetricians and Gynecologists. Health Care for Mothers and Infants in Rural and Isolated Areas. Washington, D.C., 1978. See also O'Connell J. *Op. cit.*

75. U.S. General Accounting Office. *Op. cit.*, p. 40.

76. American Nurses' Association. Access to Prenatal Care: Key to Preventing Low Birthweight. Kansas City, Mo., 1987, pp. 27–28.

77. Mayor's Advisory Board on Maternal and Infant Health, District of Columbia. Personal communication, 1987.

78. Dana Hughes, Children's Defense Fund. Personal communication, 1988.

79. Select Panel for the Promotion of Child Health. Better Health for Our Children: A National Strategy, Vol. 1. DHHS Pub. No. (PHS)79-55071. Washington, D.C.: Government Printing Office, 1981.

80. Mayor's Advisory Board on Maternal and Infant Health, District of Columbia. Personal communication, 1987.

81. Peterson P. A Time Flow Study: Hutzel Prenatal Clinic. Detroit: Wayne State University, 1987.

82. Research and Special Projects Unit. Pregnant Women and Newborn Infants in California: A Deepening Crisis in Health Care. Summary of Hearings held March–April, 1981. Sacramento: California State Department of Consumer Affairs, 1982.

83. Kalmuss D et al. *Op. cit.*, p. 47.

84. Ross CE and Duff RS. Returning to the doctor: The effect of client characteristics, type of practice, and experience with care. J. Health Soc. Behav. 23:119–131, 1982.

85. Poland M, Ager JW, and Olson JM. Correlates of prenatal care. Paper presented at the American Public Health Associates annual meeting, Las Vegas, 1986, p. 9.
86. See, for example, Juarez Associates. How to Reach Black and Mexican-American Women. Report submitted to the Public Health Service, Department of Health and Human Services. Contract No. 282-81-0082. Washington, D.C., 1982. See also Wan TH. The differential use of health services: A minority perspective. Urban Health 2:47–49, 1977.
87. Kalmuss D et al. *Op. cit.*, p. 48.
88. Faller H. Perinatal needs among immigrant women. Pub. Health Rep. 100(May–June):340–343, 1985.
89. Kalmuss D et al. *Op. cit.*, p. 47.
90. Chavez LR, Cornelius WA, and Jones OW. Utilization of health services by Mexican immigrant women in San Diego. Women's Health 11:3–20, 1986.
91. Johnson CD and Mayer JP. *Op. cit.*
92. Klein L. Nonregistered obstetric patients: A report of 978 patients. Am. J. Obstet. Gynecol. 110:795–802, 1971.
93. See, for example, Brown MA. Social support during pregnancy: A unidimensional or multidimensional construct? Nurs. Res. 35:4–9, 1986. See also Kleinman JC, Machlin SR, Cooke MA, and Kessel SS. The relationship between delay in seeking prenatal care and the wantedness of the child. Paper presented at the American Public Association annual meeting, Anaheim, California, 1984. Chapter 3 contains additional discussion of this topic.
93a. Jones EF, Forrest JD, Henshaw SK, Silverman J, and Torres A. Unintended pregnancy, contraceptive practice and family planning services in developed countries. Fam. Plan. Perspect. 20:53–67, 1988, p. 55.
94. Poland ML and Giblin PT. Personal barriers to the utilization of prenatal care. Paper prepared for the Committee to Study Outreach for Prenatal Care. Institute of Medicine, Washington, D.C., 1987.
95. Toomey BG. *Op. cit.*
96. Bowling JM and Riley P. Access to Prenatal Care in North Carolina. Raleigh: North Carolina State Center for Health Statistics, 1987.
97. Oxford L, Schinfeld SG, Elkins TE, and Ryan GM. Deterrents to early prenatal care. J. Tenn. Med. Assoc. November:691–695, 1985.
98. Cumbey DA. Improved Child Health Project. Columbia, S.C.: Bureau of Maternal and Child Health, Department of Health and Environmental Control, 1979.
99. Johnson CD and Mayer JP. *Op. cit.*
100. Warrick L. A model for examining barriers to prenatal care and implications for outreach strategies. Paper presented at the American Public Health Association annual meeting, New Orleans, 1987.
101. Poland ML, Ager JW, and Olson JM. Barriers to receiving adequate prenatal care. Am. J. Obstet. Gynecol. 157:297–303, 1987.
102. Warrick L. *Op. cit.*
103. Poland ML. Ethical issues in the delivery of quality care to pregnant women. In New Approaches to Human Reproduction, Social and Ethical Dimensions, Whiteford L and Poland ML, eds. Boulder, Colo.: Westview Press, in press.
104. Chao S, Imaizumi S, Gorman S, and Lowenstein R. Reasons for absence of prenatal care and its consequences. New York: Department of Obstetrics and Gynecology, Harlem Hospital Center, 1984.
105. Boone M. Social and cultural factors in the etiology of low birthweight among disadvantaged blacks. Soc. Sci. Med. 20:1001–1011, 1985, p. 1008.

106. Knoll K. Barriers and motivators for prenatal care in Minneapolis. Minneapolis: Minnesota Department of Health, 1986, p. 15.
107. Children's Defense Fund. Unpublished data, 1985.
108. American Medical Association. Medical care for indigent and culturally displaced obstetrical patients and their newborns. J. Am. Med. Assoc. 245:1159–1160, 1981.
109. Scrimshaw SCM, Engle PM, and Horsley K. Use of prenatal services by women of Mexican origin and descent in Los Angeles. Los Angeles: University of California at Los Angeles, 1985.
110. Research and Special Projects Unit. Op. cit., p. 51.
111. Chao S et al. Op. cit.
112. Poland ML et al. Op. cit.
113. Drugs get choke hold in early stages of life. Washington Post, January 17, 1988.
114. Margaret Haegarty, Harlem Hospital Center. Personal communication, 1988.
115. Chavkin W, Kristal A, Seabron C, and Guigli P. The reproductive experience of women living in hotels for the homeless in New York City. N.Y. State J. Med. January:10–13, 1987.
116. Boone M. Op. cit.
117. Poland ML et al. Op. cit.
118. Giblin PT, Poland M, and Sachs B. Pregnant adolescents' health information needs: Implications for health education and health seeking. J. Adol. Health Care 7:168–172, 1986.
119. Johnson S, Gibbs E, Kogan M, Knapp C, and Hansen JH. Massachusetts Prenatal Care Survey: Factors Related to Prenatal Care Utilization. Boston: SPRANS Prenatal Care Project, Massachusetts Department of Public Health, 1988.
120. Cumbey DA. Op. cit.
121. Cogswell BE and Fellow C. Adolescents' perspectives on the health care system: A determinant of fertility. Report submitted to the National Institute of Child Health and Human Development. Contract No. 1-HDE28737. Bethesda, Md., 1982.
122. Furstenberg, Jr. FF. The social consequences of teenage parenthood. Fam. Plan. Perspect. 8:148–164, 1976.
123. Cogswell BE and Fellow C. Op. cit.

Chapter

3

Women's Perceptions of Barriers to Care

The perspectives presented in the preceding two chapters are not new. Many studies have already noted that the absence of private insurance, for example, can impede prompt enrollment in prenatal care. Not as well documented is the personal significance of various barriers to women themselves. Few reports on obstacles to prenatal care cite "consumer" views, and programs aimed at increasing participation in care are often designed without careful consideration of women's experiences in obtaining prenatal services.

To begin filling the gap, this chapter summarizes several studies that have asked women to identify factors that limited their use of prenatal services during pregnancy. The chapter also presents a brief section on obstetricians' views about factors causing late registration in care. It concludes with a synthesis of several studies that have used multivariate analysis to define the characteristics (demographic, social, attitudinal, and others) that predict insufficient prenatal care.

The Committee's interest in the consumer perspective was stimulated in part by the experience of Lea County, New Mexico, where a survey of clients concerning barriers to prenatal care helped shape a local initiative to increase early enrollment (see Appendix A for more detail). In the early 1980s, a grant from The Robert Wood Johnson Foundation supported a major effort in Lea County to reduce its infant mortality rate. Although the area reported one of the highest per-capita incomes in the state, its infant mortality rate was the highest among counties with over 1,000 births per year, and use of prenatal services among some groups in the county was very low. To determine what might account for the limited use of prenatal care, a survey of women's views about barriers to care was initiated at the request of several community physicians who felt that financial obstacles were probably unimportant and that factors such as cultural practices and lack of information were decisive. Four hundred mothers were interviewed, of whom 92 had recently arrived in labor at the area's only hospital having had little or no prenatal care. Contrary to physicians' expectations, 77 percent of these 92 women stated that they had not received prenatal care because they believed they could not afford it.[1] This significant difference between the perceptions of providers and clients helped stimulate effective remedial action.

SELECTION AND SYNTHESIS OF STUDIES

To learn more about women's views concerning barriers to prenatal care, the Committee searched for studies of women who had obtained insufficient prenatal services and who had been asked about factors they felt had caused their delay in entering care. Only studies completed in the last 10 years—preferably in the last 5 years—were reviewed. Surveys with fewer than 50 respondents were not included in the synthesis described below but were considered nonetheless for possible additional perspectives. The Committee was particularly interested in studies that surveyed three groups of women: those who had obtained insufficient prenatal care; those who had obtained no prenatal care at all; and adolescents, particularly those 17 and under.

Seventeen studies that met these criteria were located;[2–18] a few of them reported on two of the three groups. Fifteen presented data on barriers reported by women with insufficient prenatal care; six presented data on barriers cited by women who had obtained no prenatal care at all; and three studies included a special analysis of the barriers cited by adolescents. In the next three sections, each of these sets of studies is discussed.

Studies of Women with Insufficient Prenatal Care

Fifteen studies of women who had obtained insufficient care are characterized in Table 3.1* along several dimensions: the year in which the data were collected; whether the data were collected in the prenatal or postpartum period; the number of women who responded with valid data;

---

*The sixteenth study listed on Table 3.1, from Hartford, is discussed in the section on adolescents.

TABLE 3.1 Studies of Barriers to Care Cited by Women with Insufficient Prenatal Care

Study	Year Data Collected[a]	When Data Collected (PN, PP)[b]	Usable Responses to Study (no.)/Overall Response Rate (%)[c]	Measure of Insufficient Care Used in Reporting Data[d]	Women with Insufficient Care[e] (no.)	Women with Insufficient Care Who Gave Data[f] (no.)	Checklist (CL) or Open-Ended (OE) Questions
GAO; 32 communities in 8 states	1986–1987	PP, usually within 1 day; sometimes up to 2 months PP	1,159/69	Kessner's definition of inadequate care	230	Not stated; presumably about 230	CL
Johnson and Mayer; Texas	1986	PP, during hospital stay	2,032/70	Care begun in 2nd or 3rd trimester or not at all	626	486	CL
Duke et al.; Oklahoma	1986	PP, within 2 days	793/90	Care begun during 1st trimester but fewer than 9 visits, or care begun after 1st trimester	270	255	CL
Mertens; Illinois	1984–1985	PP (not further defined)	4,723/29	Care begun after 1st trimester	1,174	1,174	CL
Learner et al.; South Carolina	1986	PP, in first few days	1,076/80	5 or fewer visits or care begun in 3rd trimester, or both	136	130	CL
Swink; Oklahoma Memorial Hospital	1984	PP, within 72 hours	206/52	3 or fewer visits	103	103	CL
Johnson et al.; Massachusetts	1986	PP, 7 to 10 months	2,587/84	Kessner's definition of inadequate care	443	443	CL
Toomey; Ohio	1983–1984	PN	2,444/80	Care begun after 1st trimester	1,373	NA	CL
Beatly; Denver	1985	PN and PP, within 3 days	265/NA	Care begun after 1st trimester	134	134	CL

Study; Location	Year[a]	Timing[b]	Response[c]	Measure[d]			Type
Chao et al.; New York City	1977	PP, within 2 days	474/NA	Not registered for prenatal care in hospital where delivered	220	220	OE
Oxford et al.; Memphis	1984–1985	PN	101/NA	Care begun in 3rd trimester	47	NA	OE and CL
Lake and Nixon; Hillsborough County, Florida	1985	PP, within 2 days	104/NA	1–8 visits	53	36	OE
Kalmuss et al.; New York City	1985–1986	PP, within several days	568/73	Recalled difficulty obtaining care at first provider site approached	63	63	OE
Bowling and Riley; North Carolina	1985	PP, up to 19 months	551/46	Kessner's definitions of intermediate and inadequate care	333	333	OE
Imershein et al.; Florida	1987	PP, up to 12 months	986/98	Care begun in 3rd trimester or not at all	566	445	OE
Christison-Lagay and Crabtree; Hartford, Connecticut	1982	PN	245/NA	Later registration in prenatal care	NA[g]	NA[g]	CL

[a] The year or years in which data were collected usually correspond to the year or years in which the women surveyed gave birth.
[b] PN, prenatal; PP, postpartum.
[c] The response rate is calculated by dividing the number of usable responses received into the number of questionnaires distributed or interviews attempted. For case-control studies, the response rate refers to the percentage of cases used in the analyses out of all those meeting study criteria.
[d] See Chapter 1 for a more detailed discussion of measures of prenatal care.
[e] The number of women with insufficient care whose responses were usable.
[f] The actual number of women for whom data on barriers to care were reported by the investigators.
[g] Women were interviewed during their prenatal visits, and the factors associated with relatively earlier or later registration in care were studied using a card-sort process. There was no attempt to define a subset of women with insufficient care.

the overall response rate; the study's definition of insufficient prenatal care; the number of women with insufficient care who provided data regarding barriers to care; and whether the information on barriers was obtained through open-ended questioning or a self-administered checklist.

To synthesize the results of these studies, they were analyzed in two groups: those that used a self-administered checklist (nine studies) and those that used open-ended questions (six studies). First, the comparability of the nine checklists was assessed. To help in this content analysis, 10 broad categories were defined into which all of the individual checklist items could be fitted. The eleventh category was for the few items that could not be otherwise classified. Table 3.2 shows the items that were subsumed within each category. The checklists were then analyzed again to determine which categories were on each list. This step was necessary to avoid pooling results from checklists that may have had nonequivalent contents. Finally, the top four barriers cited by the women were identified for each survey.

Table 3.3 presents the results of analyzing the nine checklist studies. It compares the lists' contents and notes the top four barriers reported by each (see the footnotes to the table). As the table shows, all checklists included items on financial obstacles to care and on transportation problems. Eight of the nine included prenatal care being poorly valued, some measure of inhospitable institutional practices, and a dislike or fear of prenatal care. Many of the other five categories were also covered by a majority of the nine surveys.

To summarize the six studies that used open-ended questions, responses were assessed using the same 10 categories, and the four most frequently cited barriers were noted. Because open-ended questions by definition do not present respondents with a checklist or similar form to complete, the process for analyzing content described above was not necessary. Table 3.4 presents the responses recorded in these six studies.

Both data sets (Tables 3.3 and 3.4) reveal that financial barriers—particularly inadequate or nonexistent insurance and limited personal funds—are the most important obstacles reported by women who received insufficient care. Transportation emerged as a substantial barrier in the checklist studies, although, as noted in Chapter 2, this barrier should probably be viewed primarily as a proxy for general financial stress rather than as a separate obstacle.

A very important message from both types of studies is that many women who obtain insufficient care attach a low value to prenatal care. This barrier was second only to financial problems in the open-ended studies and was in third place in the checklist studies. Other barriers that frequently appeared in both types of surveys among the top four include some variation on "I didn't know I was pregnant," and inhospitable institutional practices. The open-ended questions also reveal that limited

TABLE 3.2 Items Included in Each of the 11 Categories of Barriers to Care Cited by Women with Insufficient Prenatal Care[a]

1. *Financial*
   Not enough money
   Couldn't afford it
   No insurance
   Insurance didn't cover prenatal care
   Cost of the visit
   Not eligible for Medicaid
   Problems with Medicaid
   Financial, not further specified

2. *Transportation*
   Couldn't find a way to get to the appointment
   No transportation
   Transportation, not further specified

3. *Prenatal care poorly valued or understood*
   Already knew I was pregnant, so no reason to go
   Prenatal care is not necessary
   It's not important to seek prenatal care early
   I felt fine so there was no reason to come in earlier
   Prenatal care is necessary only if you're feeling sick
   I already knew what to do since I had been pregnant before
   I had no problem in previous pregnancies, so I didn't need to come
   Friends and relatives could answer my questions
   Too busy
   Too many other problems/things to do
   No room in my schedule

4. *Didn't know I was pregnant*
   I was not aware I was pregnant
   I didn't realize I was pregnant for a long time

5. *Negative institutional practices*
   Wait in office too long
   Too much paper work involved
   Clinic hours inconvenient
   Could not miss work
   Could not get time off from work
   Language problems
   No one spoke my language well enough
   Location inconvenient

Continued

[a]The wording of each item included under the 11 major headings is either that used in an individual study or a synthesis of very similar items from several studies.

TABLE 3.2 *Continued*

I didn't know where to go
I was new in town and didn't know where to go
I didn't know about the clinic

6. *Ambivalent/fearful about being pregnant*
   I changed my mind about wanting an abortion
   I didn't think about being pregnant
   I was afraid to find out I was pregnant
   I did not want others (parents, friends) to know I was pregnant
   I didn't want to tell others I was pregnant

7. *Limited provider availability*
   No doctors, nurses, or midwives in the area
   My regular doctor did not provide prenatal care
   I was turned away from the first place I tried to get care
   No doctor would see me
   The doctor/clinic was not taking new patients
   Could not get an appointment at all
   Could not get an appointment earlier
   Couldn't find a doctor who took Medicaid patients

8. *Child Care*
   No one to take care of my children (or other family members)
   Problems arranging child care
   Child care, not further specified

9. *Disliked/scared of/dissatisfied with prenatal care/provider*
   Disliked or scared of doctors, medical tests and procedures
   Previous poor experience with health clinics
   Don't like the provider or provider's behavior
   Never see the same doctor twice
   Dissatisfied with prenatal care, not further specified

10. *Other fears*
    I was afraid I'd be asked to have an abortion
    I was afraid they would take my baby away
    Immigration problems
    I was afraid I'd be reported to the INS (Immigration and Naturalization Service)
    I was afraid, not further specified

11. *Other reasons*
    Family problems
    My family didn't want me to go
    Was not in the area until time of delivery

TABLE 3.3 Four Most Frequent Barriers to Care, Rank Ordered, Cited by Women with Insufficient Prenatal Care, Checklist Questions

	Study									Studies That Included Item (no.)	Studies with Item in Top Four	
Barrier	GAO; 32 Communities in 8 States	Johnson and Mayer; Texas	Duke et al.; Oklahoma	Mertens; Illinois	Learner et al.; South Carolina	Swink; Oklahoma Mem. Hospital	Johnson et al.; Massachusetts	Toomey; Ohio	Beatly; Denver		No.	%[a]
Financial	1	1	1,2	1	1	1	1,2	1,3	2	9	9	100
Transportation	3[b]	3[b]	3	3	2	2	4	4	PN	9	8	88
Prenatal care poorly valued	3[b]	2	PN	NC	PN	3[b]	PN	PN	1	8	4	50
Didn't know pregnant	2	PN	NC	NC	4	NC	PN	PN	3	6	3	50
Negative institutional practices	PN	3[b]	PN	NC	3	3[b]	PN	2	PN	8	4	50
Ambivalent/fearful about pregnancy	PN	NC	NC	NC	PN	NC	3	PN	4	5	2	40
Limited provider availability	PN	PN	PN	4	PN	NC	PN	PN	NC	7	1	14
Child care	PN	PN	4	NC	PN	PN	PN	PN	NC	7	1	14
Dislike/scared of prenatal care	PN	PN	PN	NC	PN	PN	NC	PN	PN	8	0	0
Other fears	PN	PN	NC	NC	NC	NC	NC	PN	NC	3	0	0
Other reasons	NC	PN	NC	2	NC	NC	NC	NC	NC	2	1	50

NOTES: PN indicates item was present on the checklist but was not one of the four barriers most frequently cited. NC indicates item was not on checklist.

[a]Obtained by dividing the number of studies with the item in the top four by the number of studies that included the item.
[b]Tied items.

TABLE 3.4 Four Most Frequent Barriers to Care, Rank Ordered, Cited by Women with Insufficient Prenatal Care, Open-Ended Questions

| Barrier | Study | | | | | | Studies with Item in Top Four (%) |
	Chao et al.; New York City	Oxford et al.; Memphis	Lake and Nixon; Hillsborough County, Florida	Kalmuss et al.; New York City	Bowling and Riley; North Carolina	Imershein et al.; Florida	
Financial	1,2	1[a]	2	1	2	1,2	100
Transportation			3		1	3	50
Prenatal care poorly valued	3[a]	1[a]	1,4				66[b]
Didn't know pregnant				3	3		33
Negative institutional practices				4	4[a]		33
Ambivalent/fearful about pregnancy							0
Limited provider availability				2	4[a]	4	50
Child care							0
Dislike/scared of prenatal care		2					16
Other fears							0
Other reasons	3[a]	3					33

[a]Tied items.
[b]Because item appears twice among first four barriers in one study, the item is counted one extra time in computing the figure for the last column.

provider availability and dislike or fear of prenatal care are important obstacles. These data suggest that removing financial impediments to care would be a highly appropriate response to the views of women themselves, as would efforts to combat the opinion that prenatal care has little or no value.

Studies of Women with No Prenatal Care

Six surveys analyzed barriers reported by women who obtained no prenatal care at all, a group widely recognized as being at high risk for numerous social and medical problems (see Table 3.5). These surveys are characterized in the table by the same variables used to describe the surveys of women with insufficient care. As before, the studies were analyzed in two groups—those that used checklists versus those that used open-ended questions.

Again, financial barriers emerge as the most important obstacle (Table 3.6). In five of the six surveys, financial problems were the most frequently cited barrier. The second was a low valuation of prenatal care, a finding which suggests that many women who have received no prenatal care are particularly isolated from health services generally and may have only limited appreciation or knowledge of their value. It is also consistent with the view that these women live complicated, highly stressful lives characterized by many daily problems and struggles (see quotation below). It is perhaps not surprising that, for them, prenatal care is of low priority. Table 3.6 also reveals that other commonly reported barriers include transportation difficulties, inhospitable institutional practices, and a dislike or fear of prenatal services.

These studies of women with no prenatal care at all are a rich source of data and descriptive material. In their study of high-risk New York City neighborhoods, for example, Kalmuss et al. summarized a range of demographic, behavioral, and attitudinal variables that distinguished women who had received some prenatal care from those who had obtained none. They found that:

... women who reported receiving no prenatal care during their pregnancies are more likely to be disadvantaged socioeconomically [than a comparison group of women who received at least some care]. They are more likely to be single mothers and to have left high school before graduation. The no care women are behind other women educationally. Only 35 percent of them had the appropriate number of years of schooling for their age group, as compared to 60 percent of the total sample. Perhaps because of poverty and low levels of education, the no care women at best were peripherally connected with the health care system. They were significantly less likely to have a regular health care provider, to have received prenatal care in a previous pregnancy, or to be insured. The attitudes expressed by these women regarding health

TABLE 3.5 Studies of Barriers to Care Cited by Women with No Prenatal Care

Study	Year Data Collected[a]	When Data Collected (PN, PP)[b]	Usable Responses to Study (no.)/ Overall Response Rate (%)[c]	Women with No Care (no.)	Women with No Care Who Gave Data (no.)	Checklist (CL) or Open-Ended (OE) Questions
Richwald et al.; Los Angeles	1987	PP, during hospital stay	251/77	251	251	CL
Kalmuss et al.; New York City	1985–1986	PP, within several days	568/73	85	851	OE
Johnson and Mayer; Texas	1986	PP, during hospital stay	2,032/70	NA	81	CL
Chao et al.; New York City	1977–1978	PP, within 2 days	474/NA	42[d]	42	OE
Bowling and Riley; North Carolina	1986	PP, up to 19 months	551/46	218	218	OE
Imershein et al.; Florida	1987	PP, up to 12 months	986/98	246	246	OE

[a]The year or years in which data were collected usually correspond to the year or years in which the women surveyed gave birth.
[b]PN, prenatal; PP, postpartum.
[c]The response rate is calculated by dividing the number of usable responses received into the number of questionnaires distributed or interviews attempted. For case-control studies, the response rate refers to the percentage of cases used in the analyses out of all those meeting study criteria.
[d]A few of the respondents may actually have received some prenatal care.

TABLE 3.6 Four Most Frequent Barriers to Care, Rank Ordered, Cited by Women with No Prenatal Care, Checklist (CL) and Open-Ended (OE) Questions

	Study						
Barrier	Richwald et al.; Los Angeles (CL)	Johnson and Mayer; Texas (CL)	Kalmuss et al.; New York City (OE)	Chao et al.; New York City (OE)	Bowling and Riley; North Carolina (OE)	Imershein et al.; Florida (OE)	Studies with Item in Top Four (%)
Financial	1	1	3	1,2	1	1,2	100
Transportation	PN	2			3	3	50
Prenatal care poorly valued	3	3	1,4[a]	3[a]			83[b]
Didn't know pregnant	NC	PN			2		CC
Negative institutional practices	2	4				4	33
Ambivalent/fearful about pregnancy	NC	NC	2				CC
Limited provider availability	PN	PN			4		16
Child care	4	PN					16
Dislike/scared of prenatal care	PN	PN	4[a]	3[a]			33
Other fears	PN	PN					0
Other reasons	PN	PN					0

NOTES: PN indicates item was present on the checklist but was not one of the four barriers most frequently cited. NC indicates item was not on checklist. CC indicates percentage cannot be computed because one or both checklists did not contain the item.

[a]Tied items.

[b]Because item appears twice among first four barriers in one study, the item is counted one extra time in computing the figure for the last column.

care in general or prenatal care specifically reflect their marginal connection with health services. Women who received no prenatal care held negative attitudes toward health care; they were late in recognizing their pregnancies; and a third of them believed that if a woman feels fine there is no need for her to seek prenatal care. They were also likely to report several difficulties obtaining prenatal care, and to worry that doctors or nurses might tell them 'to stop doing some things' she [sic] likes to do. A final manifestation of the plight of these women is their rate of drug use, [which was] over three times the rate of reported drug abuse in the total sample. While high, this rate of reported drug abuse among no care women may be an underestimate. Given the strong social sanctions regarding drug use during pregnancy, it may only be women with the strongest dependencies who are detected or who give a self-report.[19]

It should be noted that many of these studies of women with no prenatal care (and of women with insufficient care as well) were conducted before the current increase in drug use associated with "crack" became evident. If these surveys were repeated in 1988, drug use might emerge as a more prominent reason for insufficient use of prenatal care, and particularly for lack of care altogether, although drug-abusing women may not readily admit their habit.

Richwald et al.[20] and Kalmuss et al.[21] asked women with no care if they had actually tried to get care. Forty percent and 27 percent of the two samples, respectively, reported that they had not, which is consistent with the low value they report attaching to prenatal services and, perhaps, with their expectation of encountering difficulties in obtaining care. Conversely, 60 percent and 73 percent of the two groups stated that they *had* tried to get care, a finding that underscores the power of the other barriers.

Though not based on direct questioning of women, and thus not included in Tables 3.5 and 3.6, the research of Joyce merits mention here.[22] She examined the records of 70 women who had obtained no prenatal care. Notes in these medical records confirmed the importance of internal barriers such as depression, denial, and fear. She concluded that, for this sample of women, psychosocial issues were greater barriers to care than such external obstacles as lack of insurance or transportation problems.

The picture that emerges from these sources is of a group of women with multiple problems and obstacles that stand between them and prenatal services. Financial problems, social isolation and disorganization, and a low priority accorded prenatal care compound one another, resulting in a failure to receive any prenatal supervision at all. Perhaps even more so than for women with insufficient care, it is unlikely that any single corrective step, such as removing financial barriers to care, would solve all the access problems for members of this group. The data suggest that a variety of interventions are needed, aimed as much at basic social functioning as at economic status.

Studies of Adolescents

The Committee reviewed three studies that assessed teenagers' views of barriers to prenatal care: the Massachusetts and South Carolina prenatal care surveys and a study conducted in Hartford, Conn.[23] All three are described in Table 3.1. Both statewide surveys used checklists to inquire about barriers to care; as noted in Table 3.3, the checklists were very similar. The Hartford study used a card-sort process to help the teenagers rank the importance of various obstacles.

The Massachusetts survey reported on 302 teenagers age 19 and younger. In descending order, the top four barriers that these young women reported were no health insurance or not enough money to pay for care, fear of doctors and medical procedures, ambivalence about the pregnancy, and denial. This survey did not cross-tabulate the data on barriers with the actual amount of prenatal care received by the respondents.

The South Carolina survey included 63 teenagers age 17 and younger who were asked about problems obtaining prenatal care. In descending order, the four most common barriers cited were lack of money or insurance, lack of transportation, problems scheduling an appointment, and long waiting times in clinics. This study also did not cross-tabulate barriers data with amount of prenatal care.

The 1983 Hartford survey of 245 women included 73 teenagers, pregnant for the first time and under age 18 at the time of conception. About a third of these teenagers entered prenatal care in the first trimester of pregnancy, the rest in the second or third. A card-sort process showed that such factors as denial, fear of parental reaction, shame, and fear of being seen in a clinic were the most significant barriers to obtaining earlier prenatal care. Such other barriers as financial problems or lack of knowledge about how to enter the health care system were not as important. The authors point out, however, that costs may not have emerged as an important barrier because "prenatal care in Hartford is free for Hartford residents. No one is required to bring cash to any visit nor is a bill sent."[24]

These three studies suggest that both personal and financial issues are major concerns for adolescents, as they are for many older women. But for the younger women such internal factors as fear, shame, and denial may well overshadow financial obstacles, at least at the outset. Given their youth, adolescents may also be particularly likely to know little about prenatal care and to place a low value on what they do know of it. Common sense suggests that when adolescents actually try to seek care, the problems of limited personal funds and no insurance also loom large. Teenagers are particularly unlikely to have the personal resources to pay for care themselves, and if an adolescent has private health insurance as a family dependent, the policy may exclude coverage for her prenatal care.

The problems an adolescent may face in using Medicaid to finance prenatal care are described in Chapter 2.

Limitations

The limitations of these studies in understanding barriers to prenatal care include the following:

a. Sample sizes are often small, limiting the ability to generalize findings to larger groups of women or to conduct careful statistical analysis.

b. Sampling strategies are not always methodologically sound. Convenience samples and other nonrandom approaches are common. Selection bias is present in most.

c. Few have been published in peer-reviewed journals or elsewhere, which may reflect their overall quality.

d. Checklists may not allow women to account accurately for the subtle and complicated issues that influenced their use of prenatal care.

Despite these limitations, it is evident that asking women themselves why they did not receive sufficient prenatal care has merit. The clear, common themes that emerge from these personal perspectives reinforce the information on barriers to care presented in Chapter 2. The studies also provide a rich source of data that program planners can use in designing actions to improve use of prenatal care. Although some communities may need to conduct additional surveys to gain a more refined understanding of barriers to care, the studies summarized in this chapter are already highly informative and form a basis for action.

PROVIDER PERSPECTIVES

Do providers of prenatal services see barriers to care in roughly the same way their clients do? In a 1987 survey by the American College of Obstetricians and Gynecologists, 2,400 of the college's members were asked to review and rate a list of 11 potential explanations for late registration in prenatal care. The items, similar to those in the client surveys just summarized, are listed below; the percentage of respondents who ranked the reason as "very important" is given in parentheses:

1. Cannot pay for prenatal care/do not have insurance or Medicaid (53 percent)
2. Don't think prenatal care is necessary (42 percent)
3. Difficulties with transportation (37 percent)
4. Inadequate child care (25 percent)
5. Fear of doctors, medical examinations, clinics, hospitals (23 percent)

6. Don't know where to get prenatal care (20 percent)
7. Frustration with the waiting time for individual appointments (20 percent)
8. Long waiting list for a first appointment (19 percent)
9. Cannot arrange time off from work for prenatal appointments (14 percent)
10. Afraid of arrest or deportation if illegally in this country (10 percent)
11. Cultural bias against male providers (5 percent)

The age and sex of the respondent, type of practice, whether or not the provider cared for any Medicaid patients, and size of the community in which he or she practiced influenced the ranking of the reasons. For example, 46 percent of providers who offer prenatal care to Medicaid patients ranked the reason "don't think prenatal care is necessary" as very important, versus 37 percent of those who do not see Medicaid patients. Female obstetricians ranked transportation, child care problems, long waiting times to obtain appointments, and long waits in offices or clinics themselves as more important barriers to care than did male obstetricians. Younger providers found more items to be important barriers to care than older ones. In general, however, virtually all respondents agreed that three barriers are the most significant—financial problems, a low value attached to prenatal care, and transportation problems.[25] Thus, there is notable agreement between clients and obstetricians.

MULTIVARIATE ANALYSIS

Multivariate analysis of factors associated with insufficient prenatal care can help bring some order to the voluminous data on obstacles to care. Studies using this approach typically pool the many characteristics that seem to distinguish women who have had adequate prenatal care from those who have not (demographic, psychological, attitudinal, self-reported barriers, and so on) and ask which factors best predict level of care when all factors are considered simultaneously. As such, these studies consider the combined effect of the demographic factors described in Chapter 1, the barriers to care outlined in Chapter 2, and the perceptions of women regarding barriers described above. Table 3.7 lists 12 studies that have used multivariate analysis to determine predictors of prenatal care use[26–31] and characterizes each study along a variety of dimensions. (Some of these studies also reported results of direct questioning of clients and were therefore included in the preceding discussion.)

Because few of the 12 studies listed all of the items entered into the multivariate analysis, it is not possible to pool results. Also, many studies

TABLE 3.7 Multivariate Analyses of Predictors of Prenatal Care Use

Study	Year Data Collected[a]	When Data Collected (PN, PP)[b]	Usable Responses to Study (no.)/ Overall Response Rate (%)[c]	Subjects (no.)	Measure of Prenatal Care	Distribution of Subjects by Care Categories (%)	Type of Multivariate Analysis
Duke et al.; Oklahoma	1986	PP, within 2 days	785/90	785	Adequate—9 or more visits and care begun in 1st trimester; Inadequate—care begun in 1st trimester but fewer than 9 visits; care begun after first trimester	Adequate, 62; Inadequate, 38	Logistic regression
Johnson et al.; Massachusetts	1986	PP, 7 to 10 months	2,587/84	2,587	Kessner index	Adequate, 66.5; Intermediate, 5.5; Inadequate, 18.0	Ordinal logistic regression
Poland, et al.; Detroit	1986	PP, 1 to 5 days	111/NA	111	Slightly modified Kessner index	Adequate, 31.5; Intermediate, 31.5; Inadequate, 17.0; No care, 20.0	Stepwise linear multiple regression
Bowling and Riley; North Carolina	1986	PP, up to 19 months	551/46	551	Kessner intermediate and inadequate combined; no care	Intermediate/ inadequate, 60; No care, 40	Logistic regression
Learner et al; South Carolina	1986	PP, within a few days	1,076/80	NA	Adequate—6 or more visits and care begun before 3rd trimester; Inadequate—5 or fewer visits, care begun in 3rd trimester, or both	Adequate, 88; Inadequate, 12	Logistic regression

Swink; Oklahoma Memorial Hospital	1984	PP, less than 72 hours	206/52	203	Adequate—8 or more visits and care begun by 20th week Inadequate—3 or fewer visits	Adequate, 50 Inadequate, 50	Logistic regression
Kalmuss et al.; New York City	1985–1986	PP, within several days	568/73	NA	Trimester of registration for care	First, 26.9 Second, 27.6 Third, 30.0 No care, 14.9	Ordinary least squares regression
Warrick; Maricopa County, Arizona	1984	PP, 5–12 months	319/50[d]	319	Adequate—5 or more visits and registration before 3rd trimester Inadequate—zero to 4 visits or registration in 3rd trimester	Adequate, 66.6 Inadequate, 33.3	Stepwise discriminant analysis
Durrik and Leonardson; South Dakota	1985	PP, not further specified	150/40	150	Adequate—5 or more visits or care begun before 3rd trimester Inadequate—fewer than 5 visits or care begun in 3rd trimester	Adequate, 50 Inadequate, 50	Discriminant analysis

Continued

NOTE: NA indicates data not available.

[a]The year or years in which data were collected usually correspond to the year or years in which the women surveyed gave birth.

[b]PN, prenatal; PP, postpartum.

[c]The response rate is calculated by dividing the number of usable responses received into the number of questionnaires distributed or interviews attempted. For case-control studies, the response rate refers to the percentage of cases used in the analyses out of all those meeting study criteria.

[d]This response rate is for a slightly different sample than that used in the multivariate analysis; it is nonetheless approximately accurate.

TABLE 3.7 Continued

Study	Year Data Collected[a]	When Data Collected (PN, PP)[b]	Usable Responses to Study (no.)/overall Response Rate (%)[c]	Subjects (no.)	Measure of Prenatal Care	Distribution of Subjects by Care Categories (%)	Type of Multivariate Analysis
McDonald and Cobrun;							
Wisconsin	1985	PP, not further specified	1,198/62	859	Month care begun[e]	NA	Ordinary least squares regression
Maine	1983	PP, not further specified	1,894/48	1,518	Month care begun[e]	NA	Ordinary least squares regression
Texas	1984–1985	PP, not further specified	1,052/32	652	Month care begun[e]	NA	Ordinary least squares regression
Colorado	1985	PP, not further specified	893/37	758	Month care begun[e]	NA	Ordinary least squares regression
Pamuk, et al.; United States	1982–1983	PP[f]	7,969/79	2,158	Adequate—care begun in 1st trimester and continued at least once/month until delivery. Inadequate—care begun after 1st trimester	Adequate, 64 Inadequate, 36	Logistic regression
Imershein et al.; Florida	1987	PP, up to 12 months	986/98	565	Early—care begun in 1st trimester. Late—care begun in 3rd trimester	Early, 71 Late, 29	Discriminant analysis

[e]Three measures of prenatal care were used in this study: month prenatal care begun, ratio of actual number of visits to "prescribed" number, and Kessner index.

[f]Interviews for the 1982 National Survey of Family Growth were conducted between August 1982 and February 1983. Natality questions concerned all births between January 1979 and the date of the interview.

constructed unique scales to measure various factors thought to predict use of prenatal services (for example, scales of attitudes toward health care and of personal and family stress), which also makes it difficult to synthesize findings.

The items found by each study to predict insufficient prenatal care are presented in Table 3.8; the wording and specificity of the items have been simplified for comprehensibility. Where available, odds ratios are presented, as is the amount of variance accounted for by the items listed (r^2 value). Only items statistically significant at $p \leq .05$ are presented.

Even without pooled results, several themes are clear. First, a striking number of studies found various markers of poverty (especially inadequate or nonexistent insurance) to be significant in predicting insufficient care. The fact that the *presence* of Medicaid is also frequently found to be predictive of insufficient prenatal care underscores an important theme in Chapter 2: that although having Medicaid is undoubtedly better than having no insurance at all for the very poor women covered, the program has clearly been unable to draw low-income women into care efficiently and early in pregnancy.

Second, among most of the studies, minority status was notably absent among the factors found to predict insufficient prenatal care. This suggests that it is the concentration of other risk factors among minority groups—poverty and less education, for example—that accounts for the low level of care.

Third, the significance of unintended pregnancy emerges in many of the studies. Various descriptions of this concept appear in the analyses—unwanted, unplanned, mistimed—along with such markers as delay in telling others of the pregnancy and long intervals until the woman suspected or knew she was pregnant. Although these terms and markers are different in precise meaning, it is possible to distill an overall theme: Women who clearly planned their pregnancies and who therefore anticipated and promptly detected the early signs of pregnancy were more likely to secure adequate prenatal care than women who did not.

In their analysis of the 1982 National Survey of Family Growth (included in Tables 3.7 and 3.8), Pamuk et al. noted important racial differences in the influence of pregnancy wantedness on use of prenatal care. They concluded that for white women, whether or not a pregnancy was wanted had only a small effect on adequacy of prenatal care.

Among blacks, however, a birth conceived by a woman who did not want to become pregnant (again) is considerably less likely to receive adequate prenatal care, regardless of the mother's age, number of previous births, marital status, or her financial access to care. This fact becomes particularly important when [one considers] that approximately 22 percent of births to black women fit the definition of being "unwanted" at

TABLE 3.8   Factors Found to Predict Insufficient Use of Prenatal Care in Multivariate Analysis[a]

Study	Factor	Odds Ratio	r^2	Comments
Duke et al.; Oklahoma	Less education	1.4	NA	Age and race not found significant
	Greater economic barriers to care (difficulty paying for care, more reliance on public financial support and public insurance)	0.66		
	More access barriers (transportation problems, appointment delays, etc.)	1.23		
	Mother unemployed	1.28		
	Less social support from baby's father	1.22		
Johnson et al.; Massachusetts	Unmarried	2.0	NA	Outcome measure was adequacy of prenatal care (Kessner); also trimester of registration
	Higher parity	2.1		
	Younger	1.4		
	Lower income	1.4–1.6		
	Longer interval until woman "knew I was pregnant"	NA		
	Pregnancy unplanned	1.8		
	Dissatisfied with prenatal care	1.2		Analysis controlled for socioeconomic factors; race not found significant
	No health insurance during pregnancy	2.3		
	Used hospital clinic for prenatal care	1.5		
	Had no one to care for other children	1.7		
	Had never used [this] health care site before	1.4		
	Medicaid insured	1.6		
	Less education	NA		
Poland, et al.; Detroit	Less insurance	NA	.49	Age, parity, maternal risk, and substance abuse not found significant
	Negative initial attitude toward pregnancy			
	Longer interval until pregnancy suspected			
	Less favorable attitude toward health professionals			
	Less importance accorded prenatal care			
	Delay in telling others of pregnancy			

TABLE 3.8 *Continued*

Study	Factor	Odds Ratio	r^2	Comments
Bowling and Riley; North Carolina	Not a WIC recipient	17.8	NA	Only study that found Medicaid *increases* probability of sufficient care
	Pregnancy diagnosed by neither doctor nor health department	5.48–8.17		
	Lower income (<$10,000)	2.94		
	Higher parity	0.71		
	Younger	≤1.12		
	Unplanned pregnancy	2.91		
	Not employed full-time	2.36		
	No private insurance	2.27		
	No Medicaid	1.29		
	Black	0.29		
	No regular physician	2.72		
Learner et al.; South Carolina	Greater financial burdens (lack of money or insurance or both)	2.10	.27	
	More transportation problems	2.92		
	More problems with child care	2.62		
	Later awareness of the pregnancy	2.39		
	Higher parity	2.26		
Swink; Oklahoma	Less education	0.39	.43	
	Money problems	3.49		
	Less social support	0.14		
	Longer interval since last physician visit	1.05		
	Less importance given to seeing an M.D. as soon as pregnancy known	0.17		
	Pregnancy outcome not believed to be significantly affected by prenatal care	3.73		
Kalmuss et al.; New York City	Younger	NA	.34	
	Larger number of difficulties reported in getting care			
	Less education			
	Negative attitude toward health care providers			
	Absence of insurance			
	Lower value attached to prenatal care			
	Used drugs during pregnancy			
	Fewer positive health-related behaviors during pregnancy			

Continued

TABLE 3.8 *Continued*

Study	Factor	Odds Ratio	r^2	Comments
Warrick; Maricopa County, Arizona				
Hispanic	Low perception of efficacy of care	NA	.35	
	Don't know where to go for care			
	Higher parity			
	Not living in metropolitan Phoenix			
	Unmarried			
Non-Hispanic, white	Low perception of efficacy of care	NA	.36	
	Less adequate insurance			
	Had not seen a dentist in past 2 years			
	More afraid of seeing M.D.			
	More [sic] years in the community			
Durrick and Leonardson; South Dakota	Financial loss in last year	NA	.28	
	Complications in pregnancy			
	Absence of private insurance			
	Lower income			
	Higher parity			
McDonald and Cobrun;				Outcome measure for all four state
Wisconsin	Care paid by Medicaid	NA	.13	analyses summarized here was month care begun; analyses also done using ratio of actual to "prescribed" number of visits and Kessner index
	Care paid by self			
	Pregnancy unplanned			
	Younger			
Maine	Care paid by Medicaid	NA	.096	
	Region in state			
	Care paid by self			
	Unplanned pregnancy			
	Lower income			
	Greater travel time to care			

TABLE 3.8 *Continued*

Study	Factor	Odds Ratio	r^2	Comments
Texas	Care not provided in private physician's office	NA	.26	
	Region in state			
	Less education			
	Lower income			
	Pregnancy unplanned			
	Higher parity			
	Hispanic			
Colorado	Unmarried	NA	.23	
	Region in state			
	Lower income			
	Greater travel time to care			
	Unplanned pregnancy			
	Care paid by Medicaid			
	Less education			
	Hispanic			
Pamuk et al.; United States				
White, non-Hispanic	Less insurance	NA	NA	
Black, non-Hispanic	Younger	NA	NA	
	Higher parity			
	Unwanted pregnancy			
Imershein et al.; Florida	Later confirmation of pregnancy	NA	.38	
	Use of hospital emergency room as primary source of medical care			
	Younger			
	Less education			
	Unmarried			
	Higher parity			

NOTE: NA indicates data not available.

[a]Only factors significant at p $\leq$ .05 are recorded.

conception compared to only 8 percent of births to white women. The difference between the two race groups with respect to both the degree of unwanted childbearing and its consequences for obtaining adequate prenatal care is striking and seems to imply differing degrees of access to or use of effective birth control and/or resort to abortion when an unwanted pregnancy does occur.[32]

It is important to add that the data set used in this analysis does not permit one to control for socioeconomic status. In one study that did hold socioeconomic status constant (a study of very poor women in Harlem), intendedness of pregnancy bore no statistically significant relationship to early enrollment in prenatal care.[33]

Fourth, multivariate analysis seems to confirm a finding from the direct interviews of women, noted above: a major obstacle to enrolling some women in care is their view that it is of limited value or, perhaps more accurately, that other concerns are more important. These studies also suggest that women who secure insufficient prenatal care are less well linked to the health care system overall and report more negative attitudes toward health care providers.

Finally, the prominence of parity is noteworthy. Although many women obtain prenatal care for the first or second pregnancy, they may not do so for later pregnancies. Problems with child care, finances, and other family responsibilities may account for this trend. Perhaps, after a few pregnancies, a woman feels she understands the likely course of events, intending to seek care only if she detects a developing problem. Earlier experiences with prenatal care may also have been unsatisfying; perhaps the care was poorly explained, felt to be of uncertain value, or offered in an unacceptable manner.

The multivariate analyses confirm many of the risk factors for insufficient prenatal care outlined in Chapter 1—poverty, being unmarried, under 20, higher parity, and less than a high school education. The multivariate analyses add to this list unintended pregnancy, little value attached to prenatal care, tenuous connection to the health care system, and negative attitudes toward providers. Among the vast majority of these studies, race was not found to predict insufficient care.

These multivariate studies can assist in designing programs to improve participation in prenatal care. They help to define key risk factors and therefore can be used to identify target groups. It is important to acknowledge nonetheless that there is still much that is not known about the factors that influence participation in prenatal care (as evidenced, for example, by the relatively low r^2 values shown in Table 3.8). The demographic risk factors outlined in Chapter 1, for example, are only partially helpful in defining target groups. Race, low educational attainment and young maternal age all correlate with poverty and within poor groups lose their discriminatory power. That is, even within seemingly homogeneous low-income groups, use of prenatal care can vary appreciably, demonstrating the need for more sophisticated understanding of the factors influencing this health behavior.

SUMMARY

This chapter has presented three data sets that bring some rank order to the many factors reported to limit use of prenatal care. Surveys of clients show that although many factors keep women out of care, financial burdens, particularly inadequate insurance, are indisputably the most significant. Other important barriers reported by women include limited appreciation of the need for, or value of, prenatal care and a variety of well-known barriers to access, such as difficulty obtaining transportation. Obstetricians seem to agree with clients on the relative importance of specific barriers to care. Finally, sets of factors found by multivariate analysis to predict insufficient prenatal care include many of the demographic risk factors discussed in Chapter 1—though not generally race—plus unintended pregnancy, low value attached to prenatal care, poor links to the health care system generally, and negative attitudes toward providers.

REFERENCES

1. Russel RE. The first report on the Lea County survey of women who have delivered babies while residents of Lea County during 1976–1981. Hobbs, N. Mex.: Lea County Perinatal Program, 1982.
2. Swink C. A comparative study of users and nonusers of prenatal care services. Ph.D. diss. University of Oklahoma, 1985.
3. Duke JC, dePersio SR, Nimmo KE, and Lorenze RR. Convenience Disincentives and Pregnancy Desire in Relationship to Prenatal Care. Oklahoma City: Oklahoma State, Department of Health, 1987.
4. Johnson S, Gibbs E, Kogan M, Knapp C, and Hansen JH. Massachusetts Prenatal Care Survey—Factors Related to Prenatal Care Utilization. Boston: SPRANS Prenatal Care Project, Massachusetts Department of Public Health, 1987.
5. Toomey BG. Factors Related to Early Entry into Prenatal Care: A Replication. Columbus: Bureau of Maternal and Child Health, Ohio Department of Health, 1985.
6. Mertens D. Birth Certificate Survey on Access to Prenatal and Well Child Care. Springfield: Illinois Department of Public Health, 1987.
7. Oxford L, Schinfeld SG, Elkins TE, and Ryan GM. Deterrents to early prenatal care. J. Tenn. Med. Assoc. November:691–695, 1985.
8. Johnson CD and Mayer JP. Texas OB Survey: Determining the Need for Maternity Services in Texas. College Station, Tex.: Public Policy Resources Laboratory, 1987.
9. Learner M, Stephens T, Sears JH, and Efirt C. Prenatal Care in South Carolina: Results from the Prenatal Care Survey. Columbia: Department of Health and Environmental Control, 1987.
10. Beatley S. Barriers to Prenatal Care in the Denver Health and Hospital System. Denver: Colorado Department of Health, 1985.
11. Chao S, Imaizumi S, Gorman S, and Lowenstein R. Reasons for absence of prenatal care and its consequences. New York: Department of Obstetrics and Gynecology, Harlem Hospital Center, 1984.

12. Lake M and Nixon D. A Study of Childbearing Women at a Public Hospital in Tampa. Tampa: University of South Florida, 1985.
13. Kalmuss D, Darabi KF, Lopez I, Caro FG, Marshall E, and Carter A. Barriers to Prenatal Care: An Examination of Use of Prenatal Care Among Low-Income Women in New York City. New York: Community Service Society, 1987.
14. Bowling JM and Riley P. Access to Prenatal Care in North Carolina. Raleigh: North Carolina State Center for Health Statistics, 1987.
15. U.S. General Accounting Office. Prenatal Care: Medicaid Recipients and Uninsured Women Obtain Insufficient Care. Pub. No. GAO/HRD-87-137. Washington, D.C.: Government Printing Office, 1987.
16. Richwald GA, Rhodes K, Kersey L, and Silberman IA. No Prenatal Care Study at Los Angeles County/USC Medical Center Women's Hospital. Los Angeles: University of California at Los Angeles, School of Public Health, 1987.
17. Imershein A, Meachen S, Kelley S, and Rond P. A Survey and Analysis of Barriers to Prenatal Care in Florida's Improved Pregnancy Outcome Outreach Project. Tallahassee: Center for Human Services Policy and Administration, 1988.
18. Christison-Lagay J and Crabtree BF. Barriers Affecting Entry into Prenatal Care. A Study of Adolescents Under 18 in Hartford, Connecticut. Hartford: City of Hartford Health Department, 1984.
19. Kalmuss D et al. Op. cit., pp. 72–74.
20. Richwald G et al. Op. cit.
21. Kalmuss D et al. Op. cit.
22. Joyce K, Diffenbacher G, Greene J, and Sorokin Y. Internal and external barriers to obtaining prenatal care. Soc. Work Health Care 9:89–96, 1983.
23. See Johnson S et al. Op. cit.; Learner M et al. Op. cit.; and Christison-Lagay J and Crabtree BF. Op. cit.
24. Christison-Lagay J and Crabtree BF. Op. cit., p. 28.
25. American College of Obstetricians and Gynecologists, Committee on Health Care for Underserved Women. Ob/Gyn Services for Indigent Women: An ACOG Survey. Washington, D.C., 1988.
26. See Swink C. Op. cit.; Duke JC et al. Op. cit.; Johnson S et al. Op. cit.; Learner M et al. Op. cit.; Kalmuss D et al. Op. cit.; Bowling JM and Riley P. Op. cit.; and Imershein A et al. Op. cit.
27. Warrick L. A model for examining barriers to prenatal care and implications for outreach strategies. Paper presented at the American Public Health Association annual meeting, New Orleans, 1987.
28. Durrick SK and Leonardson GR. Profile of adequate and inadequate prenatal care persons. Pierre, S. Dak.: South Dakota Department of Health, 1985.
29. Poland ML, Ager JW, and Olson JM. Barriers to receiving adequate prenatal care. Am. J. Obstet. Gynecol. 157:297–303, 1987.
30. Pamuk ER, Horn MC, and Pratt WF. Determinants of prenatal care utilization: Data from the 1982 National Survey of Family Growth. Paper presented at the American Public Health Association annual meeting, New Orleans, 1987.
31. McDonald TP and Cobrun AF. The Impact of Variations in AFDC and Medicaid Eligibility on Prenatal Care Utilization. Portland: Health Policy Unit, Human Services Development Institute, University of Southern Maine, 1986.
32. Pamuk ER et al. Op. cit., p. 13.
33. McCormick MC, Brooks-Gunn J, Shorter T, Wallace CY, Holmes JH, and Haegarty MC. The planning of pregnancy among low-income women in central Harlem. Am. J. Obstet. Gynecol. 156:145–149, 1987.

Improving the Use of Prenatal Care: Program Experience

The previous chapters have discussed three aspects of access to prenatal care—patterns and trends in enrollment, research and anecdotal reports regarding barriers to care, and the views of women themselves about why they obtained insufficient prenatal services. This chapter pursues the question further, from a different perspective. Here, the focus is on 31 programs that have tried to improve use of prenatal care.

The chapter begins with an overview of the Committee's method of selecting programs for study and with discussion of two particularly important aspects of trying to learn from program experience—judging the quality of available data and defining what constitutes evidence of effectiveness. A five-part program classification scheme devised by the Committee is then described, and the projects studied that emphasize each approach are noted. The Committee's findings on the usefulness of the five program types for improving participation in prenatal care are then presented, and the chapter concludes with a summary of the implementation and operational problems reported to the Committee by many program leaders.

SELECTION AND CLASSIFICATION OF PROGRAMS

The Committee and staff wrote and telephoned numerous groups and knowledgeable experts, reviewed responses to a survey conducted by the Healthy Mothers/Healthy Babies Coalition, and used other methods (see

Appendix A) to identify programs that might provide data on increasing and sustaining participation in prenatal care. Because the Committee wanted its analysis to reflect the present configuration of the health care system and the many recent changes in it, the search emphasized programs currently in operation or recently completed. A few programs that have been well described in the literature were also included, even though some of them are no longer in existence or have changed significantly in recent years.

From these many sources, a master list of almost 200 projects was developed. Although the Committee believed that the list was reasonably complete at the time, it undoubtedly had omissions. In particular, ineffective programs were probably underrepresented because they are rarely described in published, or even unpublished, articles.

The Committee divided the programs into five groups, according to their major emphasis:

1. reducing the financial obstacles to care encountered by poor women through the provision of insurance or other sources of payment;

2. increasing the capacity of the prenatal care system relied on by many low-income women, which includes health department clinics, the network of private physicians who care for Medicaid-enrolled and other low-income women, hospital outpatient departments, Community Health Centers, and similar settings;

3. improving institutional practices to make services more easily accessible and acceptable to clients;

4. identifying women in need of prenatal care (casefinding) through a wide variety of methods, including hotlines, community canvassing using outreach workers or other paraprofessional personnel, cross-agency referrals, and the provision of incentives; and

5. providing social support to encourage continuation in prenatal care and, more generally, to increase the probability of healthy pregnancies and smooth the transition into parenthood.

The latter two categories include the majority of activities generally viewed as "outreach." In keeping with the Committee's charge, a special effort was made to examine programs in those categories. Of course, few programs employed only one approach, and some were quite comprehensive; nonetheless, programs were classified by what appeared to be their main emphasis.

Representatives of each of the almost 200 programs were contacted by telephone, mail, or both to learn about the program's activities and to ascertain whether they had data that could be used to judge the program's effectiveness in improving participation in prenatal care. Where possible, written reports from the programs were obtained, and in some instances program directors were asked to develop summaries of their activities and evaluation data for the Committee. These materials were used in selecting a final group of programs for more detailed study. The main criteria used in the selection process were the adequacy and quality of program data. Consideration was also given to geographic variety, to having a mix of urban and rural programs, and to including some statewide as well as smaller scale programs. The selection process resulted in a final set of 31 programs chosen for detailed analysis. Appendix A describes all 31 and includes evaluation data from each.

Only programs that were able to provide adequate descriptive and quantitative materials to the Committee by March 1988 were included in the final set of programs. Since that time, several additional programs have come to the Committee's attention, indicating that an increasing number of local communities and states are attempting to improve access to prenatal care and to determine that effectiveness of these efforts. Space and time limitations made it impossible to include these additional studies. The Committee hopes that the federal government or a private organization will continue the task begun here of collecting information on programs to improve use of prenatal care and assessing their effectiveness.

It is important to emphasize at the outset that the Committee does not view these 31 programs as model projects. Although many are innovative and some quite successful, they were chosen primarily because their data and experience were highly relevant to the Committee's task, not because the Committee saw them as standards for the nation.

In selecting these 31, it was difficult to define what constituted adequate data. The Committee had hoped to find several experimental programs with control or comparison groups that had been used to evaluate effectiveness. Unfortunately, few programs had been evaluated with any methodological rigor, and thus a compromise position had to be adopted. To be included in the Committee's review, a program did not have to have conducted a randomized clinical trial to test impact; however, it did have to be able to report such statistics as the number of women served and their trimester of initiation of prenatal care, and it had to have made an attempt to link changes in prenatal care utilization to program activities. The presence of a comparison group of some sort was considered highly desirable, even if only the before-and-after variety. Priority was given to programs for which a formal evaluation had been conducted, particularly if comparison groups were used.

The problems with such minimal criteria are obvious. For example, if a prenatal care program was in existence before a concerted casefinding and recruitment drive, the same number of women, or even more, might have been served by the program eventually without the extra effort. Or the women might have switched from a program that did not do active casefinding to the one that did, resulting in no overall increase in the number of women served in the community. In short, the absence of controls makes it difficult to tell whether changes really occurred and, if so, whether they were the result of a particular program.

A compromise position was also adopted concerning the source of program data. The Committee had hoped that there would be a substantial body of evidence available in peer-reviewed journals (or accepted for publication) to help understand program experience in improving use of prenatal care. Many programs that could shed light on this issue, however, have not published their data, and Committee staff often had to cajole program directors into releasing findings. While several published articles are included in this review, many of the descriptions are based on reports to funding agencies or documents prepared for the Committee.

As with the issues of data quality and source, careful consideration was also given to the concept of an effective program. For this review, effectiveness was defined in terms of the month of pregnancy in which prenatal care was begun or the number of prenatal visits or both. The Committee recognizes that these process measures are not as important as the outcome of pregnancy or other measures of maternal and infant well-being. As discussed in the Introduction, however, this study was limited to the narrow question of learning how best to improve use of prenatal services, taking as a given that prenatal care improves pregnancy outcome. As a consequence, programs that had assessed their impact using only birth outcome measures (such as length of gestation, birthweight, Apgar score, or infant mortality) were excluded from the final list of programs studied. A number of projects reviewed reported data on both use of prenatal care and pregnancy outcome; the Appendix, however, presents only the utilization data.

THE PROGRAMS STUDIED

In this section, each of the five program types is described in greater detail, and the 31 projects reviewed by the Committee are listed by category. Descriptive summaries and evaluation data from each program are in Appendix A.

Programs That Reduce Financial Barriers

Ample data suggest that financial barriers are a major reason why women do not seek prenatal care early or complete the recommended number of visits; this evidence was reviewed in earlier chapters. Despite the importance of financial barriers, the Committee identified very few programs that deal with them directly. Many programs try to increase the capacity of clinics frequented by low-income women, but only a few try to provide poor women with funding for prenatal care that is simple for patients to use and providers to receive and is honored in many private and public settings.

Every program identified by the Committee that takes a direct approach to reducing financial barriers is state-initiated.[1] Federal action has been limited to recent modest increases in the Maternal and Child Health Services Block Grant and gradual expansion of Medicaid's coverage of pregnant women. Unfortunately, data for evaluating both state and federal initiatives in this area are remarkably scant, as discussed later in this chapter.

Only two programs reviewed by the Committee directly confront the financial obstacles to prenatal care:

- the Healthy Start Program in Massachusetts, and
- the Prenatal–Postpartum Care Program in Michigan.

Programs That Increase System Capacity

Pregnant women who want to seek care early and keep their appointments have difficulty doing so if they live in areas with few private practitioners or publicly financed facilities, or if local providers are unwilling to accept Medicaid clients or to provide free or reduced-cost care to uninsured women. In response, many states, counties, and cities have tried to improve access to prenatal care by increasing the basic capacity of the prenatal care system used by low-income women. Initiatives include expanding existing clinic facilities, opening new ones, or paying private providers to care for uninsured women. Such efforts frequently occur in areas where services are plentiful for more affluent women, particularly those with private insurance.

This approach to increasing the use of prenatal care has a long history. The Maternity and Infant Care Projects, initiated by the federal government in 1963, often involved opening clinics where none existed or expanding existing facilities so they could accept more indigent patients. Four more recent examples of this approach were examined by the Committee:

- the Obstetrical Access Pilot Project in 13 counties in California;
- the Perinatal Program in Lea County, New Mexico;
- the Prenatal Care Assistance Program in New York State; and
- the Prevention of Low Birthweight Program in Onondaga County, New York.

Programs That Improve Institutional Practices

Access to prenatal care may also be enhanced by revising the policies and practices that shape the way services are provided. Reform of internal operations is usually achieved when the leadership of a facility concludes that it is important to make it easier for clients to obtain care or to stay in care. Improvements might include expediting registration procedures, providing interpreters, shortening the time spent in waiting rooms, offering child care and transportation, and monitoring staff courtesy.

Several examples of this approach were examined:

• two Maternity and Infant Care Projects, one in Cleveland, Ohio, and one in three North Carolina counties;
• an Improved Pregnancy Outcome Project in two counties in North Carolina;
• an Improved Child Health Project in two areas of Mississippi;
• the Child Survival Project of the Columbia Presbyterian Medical Center in New York City; and
• a perinatal system in Shelby County, Tennessee.

Programs That Conduct Casefinding

Casefinding encompasses a greater variety of activities than any of the other four approaches defined by the Committee. It ranges from very aggressive one-on-one recruiting in a neighborhood to the passive use of newspapers and posters to attract women to a facility, and from traditional referral networks to the newer concepts of hotlines and incentive programs.

Casefinding can be divided into four categories, roughly on the basis of labor intensity. The most labor-intensive activities place women—often called outreach workers—on the streets, in housing projects, in schools and welfare offices, and in other places where pregnant women may be found. These outreach workers talk with women who may be pregnant or who may know women who are. Those not receiving care are referred to an appropriate facility. In some cases, the outreach worker's task stops at that point; that is, she is responsible only for casefinding. More often, she maintains contact with the pregnant woman and provides the forms of social support described in the next section.

Hotlines, while reactive, are nevertheless quite labor-intensive, especially if their task extends beyond just answering questions. The hotlines studied by the Committee do just that. They attempt in several ways to ease the task of obtaining a prenatal appointment, to monitor follow-through, to help women arrange for other health and social services, and to encourage change at facilities that do not appear to be responding appropriately to the needs of the pregnant women referred to them by the hotline.

A third form of casefinding involves referrals or agency networking. In this approach, an organization offering prenatal services seeks referrals from other agencies with different mandates, such as housing assistance. The notion is that these other groups are likely to be in touch with pregnant women and may therefore have an opportunity to convince them of the importance of prenatal care, determine their care status, and refer women not yet receiving care to a provider. Social service and WIC agencies (that is, agencies administering the Special Supplemental Food Program for Women, Infants, and Children) are especially likely to be in touch with pregnant women and therefore be able to refer them for prenatal care. Pregnancy testing facilities and settings providing pediatric care are other potential sources of referral for prenatal care.

A fourth, relatively new form of casefinding is the use of incentives. "Baby showers" open to the public are one example, and cash or gifts for women who come to their first prenatal appointment or who keep their appointments are others. Although European evidence on the effectiveness of incentives is inconclusive,[2] several programs in the United States are experimenting with this approach.

Closely related to these four types of casefinding, and often supplementing them directly, are public information efforts to announce specific services or programs. Such activities may be sporadic or sustained over a long period of time, and they include television and radio announcements (free public service announcements or paid spots) and announcements or educational materials in large-circulation newspapers and in neighborhood newsletters, posters, pamphlets, church bulletins, and so forth. Although their effectiveness as independent forms of casefinding may be limited, common sense suggests that public information campaigns are key elements of all serious efforts to improve use of prenatal care. Target groups need to know of existing or new services, hotlines need to be advertised, clinic telephone numbers must be widely disseminated, new clinic hours must be announced, and new forms of financial assistance must be communicated to potential recipients.

It is particularly difficult to evaluate the effectiveness of casefinding activities because they are usually intertwined with such other program components as provision of free or low-cost care to poor women. Many of the casefinding projects reviewed by the Committee were able to quantify where and how they found pregnant women and to show that the women identified by the program were at high risk for insufficient prenatal care by virtue of their demographic characteristics. Very few programs, however, were able to assess whether their casefinding efforts lead to earlier registration in prenatal care (or registration at all) among the women they found; those that could were included in the Committee's review, if at all possible.

Ten examples of casefinding for prenatal care were studied:

- the Central Harlem Outreach Program in New York City;
- the Community Health Advocacy Program in New York City;
- the Better Babies Project in Washington, D.C.;
- the Maternity and Infant Outreach Project in Hartford, Connecticut;
- the Pregnancy Healthline in New York City;
- the 961-BABY hotline in Detroit, Michigan;
- the CHOICE hotline in Philadelphia, Pennsylvania;
- a free pregnancy testing program in Tulsa, Oklahoma;
- six studies that assess the role of WIC nutrition programs in recruiting pregnant women into prenatal care; and
- a Baby Shower initiative in Michigan.

The first four programs have collected data on the effectiveness of a wide variety of casefinding techniques, particularly the use of outreach workers to identify pregnant women not already in care. The next three are hotlines, and the remaining three programs find cases through cross-program referrals and the provision of incentives.

Unfortunately, no programs of general public information and education are included in this list. The Committee learned of many efforts throughout the country to alert women to the need for prenatal care and to specific services available in a particular area. However, none was able to provide adequate information on the target populations being reached or on the program's impact on use of prenatal care.

Programs That Provide Social Support

Many communities reach out to pregnant women through workers who: communicate empathetically with their clients; educate women about prenatal care, labor and delivery, and parenthood; provide referrals and follow-up on such referrals to assure that needed services are actually secured; and act as advocates for their clients in such other settings as hospitals and welfare offices. These activities have been given many names—social support, case management, patient counseling and advocacy, case coordination, and, when occurring outside a health care facility, home visiting. The services may be offered by trained social workers, public health nurses, neighborhood residents, or volunteers with various amounts of on-the-job training. The interaction may occur in the home, at a prenatal care or social service facility, in a school, or by telephone.

Social support is presumed to improve pregnancy outcomes indirectly by helping pregnant women obtain quantitatively adequate prenatal care (i.e., assisting them in keeping their appointments). Social support is also thought to improve pregnancy outcomes directly by interpreting and reinforcing provider instructions, by reducing stress through counseling and helping women become part of supportive social networks, and by educating them about nutrition, substance abuse, medications, and other topics.

Numerous projects offering intense social support have been implemented in the past few years; the following were examined by the Committee:

- the Resource Mothers Program in South Carolina (for teenagers only);
- six additional adolescent programs, reviewed as a group;
- the Prenatal/Early Infancy Project in Elmira, New York; and
- the Grannies Program in Bibb County, Georgia.

OBSERVATIONS ON PROGRAM EFFECTIVENESS

As the program summaries in Appendix A indicate, considerable time and money are being spent on these programs, and the personal dedication of their leaders is impressive. The question is whether they are working. Are women seeking care who otherwise might not? Are they seeking it earlier? Are they staying in care? When hundreds of women use a new system of care, are they women who would have sought care under the old system anyway, albeit with greater financial or other burdens? When thousands of women call a hotline and are referred to providers, would they not eventually have found providers themselves, perhaps after a more difficult search?

The answer to these questions must take into account the fact that the women who are easiest to bring into care are already in care. With each new woman enrolled, it becomes more difficult to draw women from the pool of the unenrolled. Clearly, the challenge faced by all these efforts to improve utilization is formidable.

Equally clear is that data on which to judge program effectiveness are rarely excellent and often inadequate. Most programs have no funds for evaluation; when unrestricted dollars are available, service demands usually take precedence. Even the few evaluated programs reviewed by the Committee seldom used randomization techniques or other strong research designs to assess program effects. Selection bias, in particular, clouds most evaluations. Moreover, because many programs are complex, it is often difficult to distinguish the impact of individual elements.

This is not to say, however, that no judgment can be made regarding program effectiveness. The project data summarized in Appendix A, along with numerous discussions with program staff (both in the 31 programs reviewed and in many others), have led the Committee to conclude that each of the five program types can succeed in bringing women into prenatal care early and in maintaining their participation. With a considerable commitment of resources, participation in prenatal care can be improved, whether measured by month of registration or number of prenatal visits. It is nonetheless true that the success of many programs is modest, primarily because they are anomalies in a complicated, fragmented "non-system" of maternity services characterized by pervasive financial and institutional obstacles to care.

More specific conclusions can also be drawn about the five individual program types. With regard to the first category—removing financial barriers to care—the Committee was struck by how few programs could be identified that take this direct approach to improving participation in prenatal care, despite the overriding importance of financial obstacles. As noted earlier, most try to ease financial barriers by enlarging the clinic system relied on by low-income pregnant women, rather than by enabling them to use provider systems already in place, including physicians in private practice. The Michigan initiative is unique in its legislative guarantee of access, but the Massachusetts Healthy Start Program stands out as the one that has gone the furthest in removing financial barriers to care. The financial eligibility criteria are very liberal, women can seek care from the provider they choose (if willing to accept Healthy Start clients), registration is simple, and there is no welfare stigma. The initial evaluation suggests this is a promising approach to reaching high-risk women, particularly the working poor without available cash or health insurance. Existing ties to private providers and dislike of the welfare system may make them unwilling to use a clinic and thus cause them to delay seeking care or to seek it only sporadically. The Massachusetts program seems especially well designed to overcome such problems.

The reluctance of most states to attack directly the financial barriers is unfortunate; they are the primary factor in limiting use of prenatal care. It is not surprising, however, given legislators' concern over the costs of entitlement programs. Massachusetts' experience with a provider- and consumer-acceptable and easily administered program may well lead other states in this direction.

The program data also suggest that increasing the capacity of the prenatal care systems relied on by low-income women can improve utilization among this population. Three of the four programs studied by the Committee in this category were able to provide data suggesting improvements in use of prenatal care. It is noteworthy, though, that not all were able to enlist the full cooperation and assistance of the private sector. Although some physicians in private practice can be persuaded to care for poor women through various administrative improvements in Medicaid and through other inducements, most capacity expansion is accomplished through publicly financed facilities and with the leadership of the public sector. The use of nurse–practitioners, certified nurse–midwives, and other midlevel practitioners is often central to these programs. This emphasis derives from their proven ability to work well with low-income, often high-risk clients; the probability that program costs will be less if physicians are not relied on exclusively; and the difficulty in some communities of finding physicians willing to work in public clinics or with low-income women.

With regard to the third program type—revising internal procedures and policies—the Committee found very persuasive data that such institutional modification can improve the use of prenatal care substantially. The six programs reviewed underscore the importance of the way in which prenatal care is actually organized and offered to individual women—how clients are treated, what the clinic or office procedures are, and what the atmosphere of the setting is. This is by no means an original observation—it was presented in 1976 in *Doctors and Dollars Are Not Enough*[3]—but the value of institutional self-examination has not been taken to heart in many settings. All too many anecdotes describe service policies and procedures that discourage use of prenatal care rather than facilitate it. The startling results of modifications in the method of determining Medicaid eligibility at Columbia Presbyterian Medical Center show what can be accomplished by individuals who are willing to face the possibility that "the enemy is us."

Indeed, the Committee found great reluctance to change institutional arrangements—to meddle with existing systems—as a way of increasing participation in prenatal care. It is unclear whether this hesitation is the result of negative experiences in dealing with large bureaucracies, problems in relationships between the nonphysicians who develop many of these programs and the physicians who provide the care in them, or other factors. Whatever the reason, the reluctance is clearly present. Complaints from pregnant women about long waits in clinics, rude staff, and lack of continuity of care are seldom addressed directly by the physicians in charge; more often a new facility is opened or superficial changes in clinic practices are made.

The 10 programs with data on casefinding for prenatal care—the fourth program type—presented the Committee with a wealth of data and impressions, not the least of which was the enormous creativity shown by many program leaders in devising ways to identify pregnant women and draw them into care. Interest in these programs was dampened, however, by a deep sense of unease that pervaded the Committee's assessment of them. Given the multiple financial barriers to use of prenatal care, the inadequate capacity of many existing services, and the inhospitable institutional practices described repeatedly throughout this report, the question continually arose: Casefinding for what? If care is not readily available or suited to the target population, what can casefinding hope to accomplish? How can it compensate for 6-week waits for an appointment, inaccessible clinic sites, or providers unwilling to take Medicaid clients? How can it correct the major obstacles to care that are embedded in the inadequate financing of maternity care? These issues are developed more fully in the report's conclusions and recommendations (Chapter 5). They are noted briefly here, however, because they emerged so forcefully from the Committee's assessment of the data on casefinding.

Nonetheless, the casefinding programs do offer some insights. Data from projects that conduct casefinding with outreach workers and similar personnel suggest that the number of clients recruited is often low, and cost data from the Harlem program suggest that the cost per client enrolled is very high. It is apparently not easy to identify pregnant women not already in prenatal care, particularly among the highly mobile residents of cities. Several program leaders emphasized that inner-city women are often not at home; even when they are, they are unlikely to open their doors to unknown neighborhood canvassers. They are also more likely to be victims of such other problems as drugs, prostitution, and violence, which make them unreceptive to the overtures of outreach workers. Pregnant women in rural areas, frequently isolated from others and at a considerable distance from a care facility, may be more responsive to outreach workers, but distance and inadequate communication networks limit the success of this casefinding method there as well. Nonetheless, outreach workers can sometimes find the hardest-to-reach women. Anecdotal reports from both Cleveland and Washington, D.C., suggest that periodic sweeps by outreach workers through housing projects, for example, can uncover significant numbers of pregnant women not in prenatal care. Whether these one-shot efforts lead to enrollment in care is, unfortunately, not documented.

To improve their casefinding effectiveness, many projects ask newly enrolled women how they found out about the program or who referred them. Frequently, "word-of-mouth" or "friends" are cited. Other commonly reported referral sources include cards placed in subways and buses with key telephone numbers, carefully crafted and placed radio spots, and, to a lesser extent, television spots. Program directors generally report that pamphlets, posters, and flyers are seldom cited as referral sources, although they may help to reinforce messages communicated by other means.

The hotlines give a particularly positive impression. They appear to be meeting a real need and their success shows that the telephone has great potential for casefinding. When hotlines do more than provide information and referral, when they follow-up on referrals and try to solve their callers' problems, they can help to overcome major barriers to care. The Grannies Program in Bibb County, Georgia, shows that even minimal telephone contact can improve use of prenatal care. The value of telephone canvassing as an alternative or adjunct to house-to-house canvassing (as conducted by the Better Babies Project) has only begun to be explored. Common sense suggests that this approach can have only a very small yield, but it may find some women who could not be found any other way. Of course, for women with no telephone, this casefinding method promises little help, and it is probably true that some of the women at greatest risk for inadequate prenatal care are too poor to afford a telephone.

The program data suggest that casefinding through cross-program referrals can also improve participation in prenatal care. Close ties between prenatal services and both pregnancy testing and WIC sites can lead to earlier enrollment in prenatal care.

On the negative side, the Committee found little evidence that incentives in kind or in cash brought women into care, although the amount of data available in this area is extremely limited. Programs that use this approach generally report that the women are appreciative, but program staff do not think the incentives themselves are the primary factor in initiating or maintaining care. The Committee learned that many programs are experimenting with cash payments to encourage participation in prenatal care. In a year or two, data may be available on the effectiveness of this approach.

The final category of reviewed projects emphasizes social support, principally as a means of encouraging women to continue care. Program data indicate that this approach can indeed result in an increased number of prenatal visits. Populations at greatest risk for inadequate prenatal care, such as young teenagers and low-income minority women, often require significant social and emotional support, information, advice, and caring. Those providing such assistance are well positioned to urge pregnant women to seek and remain in care and to comply with the recommendations of their health care providers. Although most programs studied in this category were for teenagers only, there is no reason to believe that the efficacy of the approach is limited to this age group.

PROGRAM DESIGN AND MANAGEMENT

The Committee noted several design and management attributes common to projects that seemed to function well and were able to provide clear descriptive and quantitative material on their activities:

• Goals were clearly defined, well understood by everyone involved in the program, and reasonable. For example, staff understood that outreach services were only one of the steps needed to improve pregnancy outcome and therefore had realistic expectations of what outreach could accomplish.

• Most program goals could be translated into a series of quantitative measures, such as trends in first trimester registration for care, and systems had been set up to track progress toward the goals.

• Similarly, program activities were carefully monitored, often through computerized systems that provide basic management information and data for program evaluation.

• The planning phase was considered important by funders and program directors and had received adequate investments of time and money. There was a shared appreciation of the need for careful definition of target populations, needs assessment, development and refinement of management information systems, and so on.

• Community residents and providers were involved in program design. Significant time was devoted to establishing strong community ties, and a high level of respect was accorded community leaders, staff from local human services agencies, and local ways of reaching consensus and effecting change.

• Involvement of the news media was encouraged to generate support, to help communicate program goals and to convey specific messages, such as the location of a new clinic site or a new source of payment for maternity care.

• Basic concepts of product marketing had been incorporated where appropriate. Program leaders understood that, in some sense, they were selling prenatal care and should therefore draw selectively on the skills of the advertising and marketing worlds.

• Particularly in community-based programs dealing with low-income women, staff recognized the multiple burdens often facing clients and the probability that such needs as employment and English-language training were more important to them than prenatal care. Accordingly, close ties with other social services were maintained, and caseworkers were responsive to competing needs.

• In programs that employed community residents in such roles as outreach worker or hotline operator, considerable resources were invested in recruitment, training, supervision, and support.

COMMON DIFFICULTIES IN PROGRAM IMPLEMENTATION AND MAINTENANCE

The Committee was struck by the amount of effort these disparate programs involve, the degree of personal dedication required of their leaders, and the difficulties many have had to overcome to make progress.

The goal of early and continuous use of prenatal care by pregnant women may seem straightforward and obviously sensible, but attaining it in the United States at present is proving to be an arduous task. Many program leaders described their struggles to implement and maintain programs. At least 14 problem areas can be defined, and, although no single program reported all of them, a discouraging number reported several. These are listed below, grouped into several clusters.

Finding Financial and Community Support

• Funds are rarely adequate to meet program goals, and persons who must raise money annually find the constant application or lobbying process exceedingly burdensome, adding worries about job security to the usual pressures of running a program. Similarly, it is difficult to sustain political and economic support for programs over many years. The attention span of political bodies is short, which creates a continuing problem of funding stability for projects that rely on public money. Several program leaders noted that, although support for "mothers and babies" receives a lot of lip service from public leaders, efforts to translate such sentiments into ongoing legislative or fiscal support often encounter great inertia. Private sector support may be somewhat less volatile, but private foundations, in particular, are reluctant to invest in a single program for many years. These problems in securing stable financing make it particularly difficult to maintain a program or to institutionalize successful pilot or demonstration programs.

• Projects that offer clinical prenatal services (as distinct from community education, for example) can have difficulty securing funding for such other program components as more intense supervision for high-risk women, prescription drugs, certain diagnostic tests, public education, casefinding, counseling, and follow-up services.

• The news media can help create and maintain broad community support for a project and can help educate women about a particular program or service. But sustaining media support can be difficult. Moreover, even if the press is willing to cover a new initiative, interest lessens as the program becomes routine, at least to outside observers. One manager noted, "It's hard to have a press conference on an old idea." Raising money for the media portion of a program is notoriously difficult. Although television and radio spots may be comparatively easy to fund early in a program, such support tends to fade as the months progress. Programs that rely mainly on public funds report particular difficulty in securing money for ongoing, high-intensity, creatively packaged media campaigns about prenatal services and reproductive health generally.

• The close relationship that many programs must maintain with area clinics, hospitals, and health departments can make it difficult for them to act aggressively on behalf of their clients in these settings. In particular, it can be awkward for a program to seek funding from a hospital or health department while simultaneously pointing out organizational obstacles to care within these institutions and advocating change.

Recruiting and Keeping Personnel

• Program managers reported that outreach workers can be difficult to recruit, train, supervise, and motivate and that only the most skilled and persistent are likely to succeed. The threat of burnout is ever present and requires specific attention and support. Program directors have found that using outreach workers effectively requires major investments of time and money and that both funders and program planners tend to underestimate the challenge posed by using them. Similarly, other service systems often have little understanding of outreach workers' roles in enhancing access to health care and often do not work well with them.

• The tasks of outreach workers may be dangerous. It is common in inner cities, for example, for outreach workers to canvass neighborhoods or housing projects only in teams or with a security guard—or both. The cost implications of such arrangements are obvious.

• Adequate money and time are seldom available for provider education about cultural and other differences between themselves and clients that may impede communication and compliance. Some programs report overt resistance to such training among providers, both those in the program and those in the community to whom program participants may be referred.

• Some program clients are hard to engage, difficult to work with, and occasionally abusive to the staff. One program manager noted: "It's hard to make the doctors and nurses like and 'reach out' to some of these women." Substance abusers in particular can put great stress on the staff.

Dealing with Bureaucracies

• Building an innovative program into an existing system is difficult and fraught with potential turf battles. Competition for space and staff positions, for computer time, for the attention of the broader organization's leadership, and for community support creates serious tensions. New programs face major bureaucratic obstacles in hiring staff; a position for the new program may be approved but cannot be filled or hiring freezes may paralyze progress altogether until ways of circumventing such obstacles are found. Differences in responsibility, autonomy, perhaps also in pay between the new program's staff and others in roughly similar positions in the existing bureaucracy can create suspicion and resentment. Worries about job security among existing staff and the discomforts of organizational change can create a chilly environment for a new program.

• Long-standing tensions between, for example, state and city health authorities, health departments and local hospitals, and physicians and nurse–midwives can interfere with programs that are trying to change the prenatal care system. One program studied by the Committee has still not been successful in employing nurse–midwives in its clinical services as originally planned because of resistance by private physicians affiliated with the major hospital in the community.

Planning and Sustaining Programs

• The start-up time of programs is often long, or at least should be long, if adequate planning and training are to be accomplished. Yet, funders are often impatient, wanting the program to begin quickly and show results soon thereafter. Long start-up periods are reported by state-level programs in particular, because they often need the tangible assistance and cooperation of multiple bureaucracies (accounting, welfare, personnel, and so on), many of which have no familiarity with maternal and child health services.

• It is hard to maintain momentum in programs dependent on high-energy founders, the charismatic people who generate fresh ideas and new programs, overcoming numerous obstacles to progress. As leaders change over time, a program's energy level often drops and the underlying rationale and essential program features can be lost. Effectiveness can also deteriorate when small, successful programs are expanded. For example, one program that began small was accepted by providers because it included a more efficient, accessible process for billing Medicaid; providers were paid promptly, and billing problems were solved relatively easily. When the program was expanded statewide, much of this billing system was lost—and provider participation along with it.

Other Problems

• The controversial issue of abortion can compromise support for prenatal programs, particularly if such programs focus on reaching women early in pregnancy. It was reported to the Committee that prenatal programs can be suspected of encouraging abortion for some clients and therefore have difficulty securing adequate support, particularly from legislative bodies.

• Low-income clients often have great difficulty finding funds for labor
and delivery; consequently, program staff must spend considerable time
helping distressed clients locate financial aid. One nurse reported that a
large proportion of her time with pregnant women is spent on this single
issue, causing considerable anxiety to both herself and the client. Other
topics such as preparation for parenthood or infant feeding options are
sometimes shortchanged in the search for financial assistance with childbirth expenses.

PROGRAM EVALUATION

The Committee also found that virtually all programs struggle with
evaluation—what to evaluate, how to build data collection into routine
program activities, how to enlist staff in the process of evaluation when
providing service is their primary focus, and, above all, how to find
adequate money, staff, and time to do high-quality evaluation studies.
Compounding such challenges is the fact that programs are often in a state
of flux. Patient populations, the number of geographic areas in which the
program operates, the nature of the services being offered—even the
forms—change frequently, making evaluation of impact difficult. Several
programs decided in mid course to study their effectiveness more systematically, but they were hampered by their late start and by the usual
resource constraints. Tensions between service goals and evaluation were
constantly evident; for example, leaders of the Resource Mothers program
reported difficulty in getting staff to adhere to certain data-gathering
routines or to such research methods as randomization. Perhaps most
troubling of all, some programs that believed they were evaluating their
activities properly were found, on closer examination, to be using inadequate evaluation designs, yielding data of limited value. The net result of
all these problems and constraints is that the quality of most program
evaluation reviewed by the Committee was poor and that considerable
energy was being wasted.

The challenge of evaluation is formidable not only for community-based
projects, but also for recent statewide efforts to reduce infant mortality and
enhance prenatal care. Illinois, California, Florida, and Connecticut, for
example, are deeply involved in efforts to improve perinatal care and infant
survival. However, the number and complexity of the interventions within
a given state, the diversity and number of settings providing the new
services, problems in collecting uniform data, the time and money required
to design statewide evaluation systems and to analyze the voluminous data
these systems generate—such problems often result in inadequate evaluation or none whatever. Maternal and child health agencies within state

health departments often have a leading role in these state initiatives, but they seldom are provided with sufficient resources to evaluate the new programs they are charged with operating.

SUMMARY

With typical American ingenuity and energy, a great variety of programs has been organized in recent years to help women gain access to prenatal care. A careful study of 31 such programs and a more limited review of many more has led the Committee to conclude that, with adequate investments of time, money, and commitment, rates of early registration in prenatal care can be improved, as can rates of remaining in care. However, many of these initiatives are only modestly successful because they are anomalies in a complicated, fragmented maternity system with pervasive financial and institutional obstacles to care. In studying these programs, the Committee noted that management and evaluation vary in quality across the programs; with regard to evaluation in particular, quality is often poor.

The Committee was particularly impressed with the effectiveness of programs that reduce fundamental financial or capacity barriers. Participation in care also can be improved through programs that try to change policies at the service delivery site so that women will feel welcomed into care, or that act as advocates for women who have encountered problems.

Nevertheless, there are some women for whom a reduction in financial barriers, an increase in service supply, and a modification in policies at the service delivery level will still not be sufficient to bring them into prenatal care early and regularly. For them, certain casefinding techniques seem particularly useful, such as cross-program referrals and hotlines. Providing intensive one-on-one social support can help to keep women in prenatal care throughout their pregnancies.

In considering all five program types together, the Committee noted that far more energy is going into outreach than into programs that reduce fundamental financial and institutional barriers, despite their importance (Chapter 2). If more programs focused squarely on eliminating basic institutional barriers, it would easier to define who the truly "hard to reach" pregnant women are and to target casefinding and social support programs more effectively.

The effort that all these programs expend in achieving even small gains is sobering. Launching new initiatives and sustaining momentum require a tremendous commitment by program leaders and funders, and many obstacles can be encountered along the way—unstable funding, bureaucratic in-fighting, private sector resistance, even physical danger. Indeed, the job of drawing more pregnant women into care seems at present an overwhelming, thankless task. As one program leader mused, "We're trying to do the Lord's work and we keep finding devils."

REFERENCES AND NOTES

1. See, for example, Petschek MA and Adams-Taylor S. Prenatal Care Initiatives: Moving Toward Universal Prenatal Care in the United States. New York: Center for Population and Family Health, School of Public Health, Columbia University, 1986.
2. Beukens P. Determinants of prenatal care. In Perinatal Care Delivery Systems, Kaminski M, Breart G, Beukens P, Huisjes HJ, McIlwaine G, and Selbmann H, eds. Oxford University Press, 1986, pp.16–25.
3. Doctors and Dollars Are Not Enough. Washington, D.C.: Children's Defense Fund, 1976.

Chapter

5

Conclusions and Recommendations

At the outset, the focus of this study was outreach for prenatal care. The Committee's charge was to determine which outreach techniques most effectively draw women into care early in pregnancy and maintain their participation until delivery. For this study, outreach was defined to include various ways of identifying pregnant women and linking them to prenatal care (casefinding) and services that offer support and assistance to help women remain in care once enrolled (social support).

Early deliberations, however, made it clear that outreach could not be studied in isolation and that the Committee's inquiries had to cover the larger maternity care system* within which outreach occurs. At least four considerations led to this expanded scope of study. First, many projects conventionally labeled outreach (that is, programs of casefinding or social support or both) were found, on closer examination, to be actively involved in such problem-solving activities as trying to help women arrange financing for an in-hospital delivery—activities that are not included in conventional understandings of outreach. Second, the goals and content of outreach programs are so heavily influenced by the larger systems within which they operate that it would have been difficult, if not useless, to analyze them apart from their surrounding environment. Third, a variety of approaches other than outreach can accomplish the goals of earlier registration in prenatal care and improved continuation in care.

---

*That is, the complicated network of publicly and privately financed services through which women obtain prenatal, labor and delivery, and postpartum care.

135

These activities include reducing financial barriers to care, making certain that system capacity is adequate, and improving the policies and practices that shape prenatal services at the delivery site. Finally, the Committee reviewed the larger maternity care system because it makes little sense to study ways to draw women into care if the system they enter cannot, or will not, be responsive to their needs. Because of this expanded scope of study, many of the recommendations contained in this chapter are directed at the maternity care system as a whole rather than only its outreach component, although specific recommendations on outreach are presented.

REVISING THE NATION'S MATERNITY CARE SYSTEM:
A LONG-TERM GOAL

The data and program experience reviewed by the Committee reveal a maternity care system that is fundamentally flawed, fragmented, and overly complex. Unlike many European nations, the United States has no direct, straightforward system for making maternity services easily accessible. Although well-insured, affluent women can be reasonably certain of receiving appropriate health care during pregnancy and childbirth, many other women cannot share this expectation. Low-income women, women who are uninsured or underinsured, teenagers, inner-city and rural residents, certain minority group members, and other high-risk populations described earlier in this report are likely to experience significant problems in obtaining necessary maternity services.

Securing prenatal services in particular can be especially difficult for these groups, as shown by the data in Chapters 1 and 2; moreover, there is evidence that utilization is actually declining among certain very high-risk groups. Recent efforts to expand eligibility for Medicaid and numerous state and local initiatives to strengthen maternity services may improve use of prenatal care somewhat, but given the modest scale of most initiatives and the magnitude of the problem, major inequities in the use of prenatal services are likely to remain. These data are deeply troubling in light of the value and cost-effectiveness of prenatal care.

Achieving major improvements in the maternity care system, particularly in the use of prenatal care, will be neither quick nor easy. Significant improvement must begin with a fundamental recognition that pregnancy and childbearing are profoundly important events requiring carefully formulated social policies and supports.

● **We recommend that the nation adopt as a new social norm the principle that all pregnant women—not only the affluent—should be provided access to prenatal, labor and delivery, and postpartum services** appropriate to their need. **Actions in all sectors of society, and clear leadership from the public sector especially, will be required for this principle to become a clear, explicit, and widely shared value.***

A consensus of this nature means that maternity services must be viewed not as a consumer good, available only to women with certain financial and personal assets, but as an essential part of the country's social and health services, comparable to public education—easily available, valued, and used by virtually all women. The merit of such social policy is amply supported by data on the effectiveness—including the cost-effectiveness—of prenatal care (see the Introduction). It is also consistent with basic civility and compassion, with the concept of adequate investment in future generations, and with the need to provide special care during a particularly vulnerable phase of life—pregnancy and childbirth. All subsequent recommendations in this report are subsumed under this one. We suggest it as a standard against which to measure a wide array of policy suggestions—ours and others'.

Attaining this goal requires major reform in the way maternity services are organized, financed, and provided in this country, particularly for low-income and other high-risk groups. Continuing to make marginal changes in existing programs is unlikely to meet the standard of universal participation that we advocate. Slowly implemented, often small expansions in Medicaid eligibility, brief bursts of publicity about infant mortality and the importance of prenatal care, efforts in a few communities to increase the number of clinics offering prenatal services—these actions, while laudable, are too limited, sporadic, and uncoordinated to overcome the pervasive barriers to care detailed in this report. Rather, the current situation dictates more purposeful action:

• **We recommend that the President, members of Congress, and other national leaders in both the public and private sectors commit themselves openly and unequivocally to designing a new maternity care system (or systems) dedicated to drawing all women into prenatal care and providing them with an appropriate array of health and social services throughout pregnancy, childbirth and the postpartum period. Although a new system might build on existing arrangements, long-term solutions require fundamental reforms, not incremental changes in existing programs.**

Several ways of designing a new system are feasible, once the political will to create one has been mustered. For example, Congress could appoint

---

*Throughout this chapter, major recommendations are bulleted (•) and in bold face; subsidiary recommendations and suggestions that develop a recommendation further are in italics.

a commission of experts knowledgeable about the maternity care system and public policy; a group of experts within the U.S. Department of Health and Human Services could be assembled; Congress could itself develop alternative proposals using existing data and opinions, drawing on the expertise of established congressional committees and such resources as the Office of Technology Assessment and the Congressional Budget Office; or an independent group could be asked for advice.

In making this recommendation, the Committee emphasizes that a commitment to enact major reforms must precede the establishment of any commission or other mechanism.* Too often, studies are funded or panels appointed without such a commitment; as a consequence, change may be postponed or fail to take place altogether.

We urge that the group chosen to work out the specifics of a new system be a technical, expert body charged only with defining the components and costs of a new maternity system, not with describing current problems yet again or with developing the political momentum needed to accomplish major changes.

Once the components of the system have been defined, action to implement the recommendations must follow; otherwise, the effort will be futile and may actually be destructive, by raising false hopes among those in need.

In recommending a new maternity system, the Committee recognizes that problems of access to maternity care are only part of the larger problem of access to health services generally. It may well be that far-reaching reforms in the overall health care system will overtake the efforts recommended here to improve access to maternity care. For example, the increasing pressures of the AIDS epidemic alone may lead to significant changes in the health care system. Nonetheless, the focus here is on maternity care, as dictated by the Committee's mandate.

Although the Committee was not asked to specify the elements of a new system or systems of maternity care, our work over the last 2 years has indicated the principles essential to significant improvement in the use of prenatal services. We presume that these same attributes would also improve the care women receive during childbirth and the postpartum period. *We urge that the new system:*

---

*This sequence was followed in the early 1980s when the Social Security system was threatened with financial difficulties. Both the President and the Congress recognized that corrective action needed to be taken and appointed the National Commission on Social Security Reform (the "Greenspan Commission") to develop a plan for solving the system's financial problems. The Commission recommended a series of measures in January 1983 and Congress adopted them later that year.

—*accommodate the maternity care needs of all women, not only women in privileged economic or geographic subgroups;*

—*embrace the full continuum of maternity services (prenatal, labor and delivery, and postpartum care), erasing the gap that currently exists between systems that provide and finance prenatal care and those that support care for childbirth;*

—*be closely coordinated with other health services used by women, improving the quality and accessibility of these related services as much as possible;*

—*offer a uniform, comprehensive package of maternity services that can accommodate variations in individual needs, as suggested by the Select Panel for the Promotion of Child Health,[1] the American College of Obstetricians and Gynecologists[2] and the American Academy of Pediatrics,[3] and the forthcoming report of the Public Health Service's Expert Panel on the Content of Prenatal Care;[4]*

—*address the liability pressures currently driving providers out of the practice of obstetrics;[5]*

—*be administered separately from the welfare system;*

—*rely on a wide array of providers, including both physicians and certified nurse–midwives, each of whom may practice in a variety of settings and systems;*

—*be financed adequately;*

—*ensure that financing mechanisms support appropriate clinical practices;*

—*include a large-scale, sustained program of public information and education about maternity care;*

—*support education and training of providers to deepen their understanding both of the obstacles women can face in securing prenatal care and their perceptions of care once enrolled;*

—*include reliable, accurate means of collecting data on unmet maternity care needs and on the performance of the new system or systems, at local, state, and national levels; and*

—*specify a structure of accountability and responsibility under the control of a federal agency, with state agencies assuming leadership.*

Many of these issues, such as the urgent need to address liability pressures, are taken up again and in more detail in later sections presenting the Committee's short-term recommendations. Here, we wish to emphasize two in particular. First, the separation of maternity care financing from the welfare system is emerging as a key element of initiatives to improve use of prenatal care among poor women, as demonstrated by recent Medicaid reforms (Chapter 2). Although Medicaid and welfare obviously need to be coordinated, the links between the two programs have had the unfortunate effect of attaching a welfare "stigma" to a health care financing program. Therefore, the notion of separating the programs administratively is important. Second, we emphasize the need for national standards of maternity care. Increased communications, rapid dissemination of new information and technologies, and increased use of national standards in malpractice suits make it ever more unreasonable for maternity care to differ widely among geographic or socioeconomic groups, although care must always accommodate variations in individual need.

It is also apparent that a deeper national commitment to family planning services and education should accompany major revisions in the maternity care system. Women with unintended pregnancies are particularly likely to delay seeking prenatal care and more than half of all pregnancies in the United States are unplanned (Chapter 2). Therefore, reducing rates of unplanned pregnancy could lead to lower rates of late entry into prenatal care. The Committee recognizes that progress in this direction is complicated and that a large literature exists on both the antecedents of unintended pregnancy and ways to reduce it. Nonetheless, a firm commitment to extending family planning services is an obvious, essential first step, particularly for those populations most at risk of unintended pregnancy (and, subsequently, poor participation in prenatal care)—low-income women, teenagers, and minorities. Such services should be easily available in numerous settings, should be provided for free or at very low cost, and should be carefully linked to prenatal services (as discussed in more detail below). High-quality, widely disseminated public information and education about family planning is also important and should be coordinated with messages about prenatal care. In fact, it might be possible to develop information and education campaigns around broad issues of reproductive responsibility and health, encompassing both family planning and prenatal care.

DEVELOPING A COMPREHENSIVE, MULTIFACTED PROGRAM: A SHORT-TERM GOAL

While consensus grows on the need for a major restructuring of the maternity care system in the United States, and while the specifics of a new approach are being defined, several more immediate steps should be taken to increase participation in prenatal care. Although some of them are quite far-reaching, they all derive from and are based on the existing maternity care system. As such, they differ fundamentally from our recommendation in the preceding section, which argues for a more profound and complete reorganization of this health care field.

• **We recommend that more immediate efforts to increase participation in prenatal care emphasize four goals: eliminating financial barriers to** care, making certain that the capacity of the system is adequate, improving the policies and practices that shape prenatal services at the site where they are provided, and increasing public information about prenatal care.

The Committee has concluded that these four reforms promise significant improvement in the use of prenatal care. The first of the four—eliminating financial barriers—is undoubtedly the most important. Indeed, we believe that if this single barrier were removed, many of the other problems noted throughout this report would decrease appreciably. Ample data indicate, however, that it is not only financial problems that keep women out of care. Other problems can impede access as well and also require attention. Thus, removing financial barriers should be viewed as a necessary—but not entirely sufficient—step in improving the use of prenatal care.

We urge that leadership for this comprehensive approach come from the federal government. Individual states and communities should not have to both develop and fund programs to improve access to care, even though some states have been particularly innovative in doing so—by offering health insurance to those with inadequate or absent coverage, for example, or by constructing new programs to supplement Medicaid and federal funds for maternal and child health. Leaving the entire task of program innovation and support up to the states is certainly consistent with political trends in the 1980s, but the federal government should nonetheless play a stronger role.

● **We recommend that the federal government provide increased leadership, financial support, and incentives to help states and communities meet the four goals we advocate. In a parallel effort, states should accept the responsibility for ensuring that prenatal care is genuinely available to all pregnant women in the state, relying on federal assistance as needed in meeting this responsibility.**

More specifically, we urge a stronger federal role in providing funds to state and local agencies in amounts sufficient to remove financial barriers to prenatal care (through such channels as the Maternal and Child Health Services Block Grant and other grant programs) and in providing prompt, high-quality technical consultation to the states on clinical, administrative, and organizational problems that can impede the extension of prenatal services. The federal government should also take more leadership in defining a model of prenatal services for use in public facilities providing maternity care; and supporting related training and research.

States should assume direct responsibility for ensuring that all women within the state have full access to prenatal services. Backed by adequate federal funds, support, and consultation, the states should invest generous amounts of time and money in extending this basic health service. This would involve states more deeply in assessing unmet needs by surveying existing prenatal services and identifying the localities and populations for which they are inadequate; contracting with various providers to fill gaps in services; and in some instances, providing prenatal services directly, through such facilities as health department clinics. In addition, the Committee suggests that each state pass legislation making the maternal and child health agency of the state health department responsible for ensuring that prenatal services are reasonably available and accessible in every community.

FINANCIAL BARRIERS

Removing financial barriers to care is the cornerstone of the comprehensive program we recommend. Surveys of pregnant women and of maternity care providers, and program experience over many years uniformly demonstrate the importance of economic circumstance—especially the presence or absence of insurance—in predicting use of prenatal services. Although expansions of Medicaid and creative state initiatives have made some progress recently in lowering financial barriers to care, the pace of progress needs to accelerate, and remaining financial obstacles need to be removed. Accordingly, as a critical first step:

• **We recommend that top priority be given to eliminating financial barriers to prenatal care.**

This broad recommendation has specific implications for all the major networks, public and private, that underwrite prenatal care. For the *Medicaid* program:

We recommend that the federal government require all states to provide Medicaid coverage of prenatal care for pregnant women with incomes up to 185 percent of the federal poverty level,* to be followed by eligibility expansions beyond 185 percent to cover more uninsured or underinsured women.

Detailed discussions of how states and the federal government can accomplish this and other expansions in Medicaid eligibility for pregnant women and other groups are contained in *Medicaid Options: State Opportunities and Strategies for Expanding Eligibility*, prepared by the American Hospital Association.[6]

---

*This is currently only an option for states (Chapter 2).

For the various *federal grant programs* (particularly the Maternal and Child Health Services Block Grant and the programs funding Community Health Centers, Rural Health Centers, and Migrant Health Centers) and for *state and local health departments:*

We recommend that federal and state authorities provide these service systems with sufficient funds to offer free or reduced-cost prenatal care without delay to all pregnant women requesting it in these settings.

Meeting this broad objective will require, among other things, more sophisticated measurement of unmet need in the areas served by these publicly financed clinics.

For *private insurance*, where coverage of prenatal care can be inadequate:

We recommend that Congress and state governments act to expand and strengthen private insurance coverage of maternity services.

This goal could be reached in various ways. For example, Congress could mandate that all employers covered by the Fair Labor Standards Act provide a defined package of maternity services to employees and their dependents. Congress could also repeal the exemption contained in the Pregnancy Discrimination Act allowing employers of fewer than 15 persons to provide no pregnancy coverage. Congress could also modify the Employee Retirement Income Security Act (ERISA) in order to permit states to require that self-funded employer health plans provide maternity benefits; more than half of employer-provided health insurance plans are self-funded and as such are exempt from state insurance regulation through ERISA.

We also urge purchasers of private insurance to press for improved coverage of prenatal care through labor union negotiations, switching to more comprehensive plans, and similar consumer-based actions. Private insurance companies themselves should take the initiative of offering comprehensive coverage of prenatal care as part of their basic insurance packages.

In all these actions, attention should be focused on eliminating such gaps in coverage as waiting periods for prenatal benefits to begin, dependent coverage that fails to include prenatal services, limited insurance for part-time or seasonally employed individuals, and burdensome copayments and deductibles for maternity services (Chapter 2).[7]

INADEQUATE SYSTEM CAPACITY

Urging all pregnant women to begin prenatal care early is a hollow message if prenatal clinics are nonexistent—or so backed up as to be nonexistent in practical terms—or if private providers are lacking or unwilling to accept low-income patients. Yet the Committee uncovered considerable evidence that capacity is inadequate in various communities, particularly for poor women (Chapter 2). Accordingly, as a companion initiative to reducing financial barriers:

• **We recommend that public and private leaders designing policies to draw pregnant women into prenatal care make certain that prenatal services are plentiful enough in a community to enable all women to secure appointments within 2 weeks with providers close to their homes.**

Methods for achieving this objective will vary across states and communities, but several approaches will probably be required simultaneously. We recommend:

—*more careful assessment at the community level of existing service capacity and of the areas and groups for whom capacity is inadequate; state leadership in this area is particularly appropriate, as noted above;*

—*more generous financing of clinic systems, in particular, to allow them to meet demand, also noted above;*

—*resolution of the malpractice crisis in obstetrics;*

—*increased Medicaid reimbursement for maternity care offered by private providers in order to increase the number of physicians who accept Medicaid patients;*

—*restoration of the National Health Service Corps and equivalent state programs to help develop an adequate pool of providers for medically underserved areas;*

—*expansion of the variety of settings in which prenatal care is offered; school-based health clinics in particular can help bring prenatal care to adolescents;*

—*increased use of certified nurse–midwives (CNMs) and obstetrical nurse–practitioners; state laws and physicians themselves should support hospital privileges for CNMs and collaboration between physicians and nurse–midwives or nurse–practitioners; eventually, large interstate variations in the laws governing the use of such midlevel practitioners should be eliminated; and*

—*leadership by the professional societies of obstetric care providers to increase the involvement of private physicians in the care of indigent women. (For example, private sector leaders should work collaboratively with Medicaid officials and leaders of maternal and child health agencies to raise reimbursement levels for maternity care, to solve administrative problems in the Medicaid program, and to develop proposals for providing physicians with incentives to serve poor women. National professional organizations should urge local ones to focus on problems of underserved women).*

The last point is particularly important. Raising Medicaid fees and addressing the malpractice problem in obstetrics are undoubtedly necessary to enhance private sector involvement in indigent care, but leadership from the professional societies is also critical. The work of the Committee on Underserved Women of the American College of Obstetricians and Gynecologists is a useful step in this regard. Other national, state, and local organizations of obstetric care providers should establish similar groups.

With regard to the specific issue of malpractice, the Committee urges public and private groups with expertise in this area to develop without delay a range of possible solutions to the current situation, perhaps experimenting with various approaches in different states. One interesting proposal is to provide sufficient funds to public agencies for them to absorb the costs of malpractice insurance for providers (MDs, CNMs, and others) who care for significant numbers of indigent women.

INSTITUTIONAL ORGANIZATION, PRACTICES, AND ATMOSPHERE

However well-organized the maternity care system appears at the state or national level, a pregnant woman experiences and judges it in her individual community, in a specific clinic or office, and with a particular provider. In reviewing initiatives to increase the early use of prenatal care, the Committee has been repeatedly impressed by the success of programs that emphasize internal institutional modification as a means of drawing more women into care and sustaining their participation. Therefore, in addition to addressing financial barriers and problems of limited capacity:

• **We recommend that those responsible for providing prenatal services periodically review and revise procedures to make certain that access is easy and prompt, bureaucratic requirements minimal, and the atmosphere welcoming. Equally important, services should be provided to encourage women to continue care; follow-up of missed appointments should be routine, and additional social supports should be available where needed.**

In this context, the Medicaid program requires special emphasis. However generous the eligibility expansions described earlier, little is gained if the task of applying for and maintaining Medicaid coverage is so difficult, complicated, and time-consuming that prompt, continuous participation in prenatal care is virtually impossible for all but the most socially organized and determined women. Accordingly:

We recommend that states shorten and simplify the process of obtaining Medicaid coverage for prenatal services and that, once a woman is enrolled, her coverage be uninterrupted throughout pregnancy, labor and delivery, and a postpartum visit.

Adopting the presumptive eligibility option and eliminating the asset test (or using a much simplified, more generous one) can help in meeting these goals, as can wider implementation of various options now available to ensure uninterrupted coverage of prenatal services (Chapter 2). Other useful steps include on-site determination of eligibility (by placing eligibility workers in maternity clinics serving low-income populations, for example), shortened application forms requiring minimum documentation, suspension of error rate sanctions in determining the eligibility of pregnant women, a single application form for several programs, and bilingual staff or interpreters.

Of course, such improvements are of little value if potential recipients know little about the Medicaid program or whether they might be eligible for coverage. Closing the gap between the number of pregnant women eligible for the program and the number enrolled requires explicit information, widely disseminated, about who is eligible and how to apply for coverage. Accordingly:

We also recommend that states and communities aggressively advertise the availability of the Medicaid program to finance prenatal care for low-income pregnant women. Materials developed for this purpose must be accurate, current, and directed to issues of pregnancy coverage and maternity services. The materials should present the information in a way that is not so complex as to intimidate potential applicants and should include clear directions about where and how to apply for the program.

Several other, more general attributes of prenatal services can also help to increase use of care and we recommend that they be widely adopted:

—services are easy to find in the telephone book, listed under several headings;
—the telephone system in an individual setting is well organized and staffed so that callers do not constantly reach a busy signal;
—reasonable efforts are made through various channels of public information to inform women of service hours and location, to advertise new maternity programs, and to alert women to services that complement prenatal care, such as the Special Supplemental Food Program for Women, Infant, and Children (WIC);
—there is a gap of 2 weeks or less between an initial call for a prenatal care appointment and the appointment itself;
—services are located near public transportation; where needed, transportation costs are subsidized or provided directly;
—a woman sees as few different providers as possible in the course of a pregnancy;

—clients spend minimal time in a waiting room (by using, for example, a staggered rather than a block appointment system);

—patients are treated courteously, not only by physicians and nurses, but also by receptionists, appointment clerks, and other gatekeepers, particularly at the first contact or visit;

—staff training is frequent and supports a positive orientation toward clients;

—careful consideration is given to women's cultural preferences, such as using female providers for women whose cultures do not accept medical examinations performed by men; similarly, health and nutrition education are consonant with cultural practices, including diet;

—adequate time is allowed for talking with clients about unfamiliar procedures and treatments;

—special efforts are made to coordinate the hours and the paperwork of prenatal services with other services needed by clients;

—appointments are timed to accommodate women's schedules, particularly those who work or go to school;

—bilingual staff or interpreters are present where common language barriers commonly exist; and

—child care services are provided or are easily accessible nearby.

PUBLIC INFORMATION AND EDUCATION

Studies of women who received insufficient prenatal care reveal that an important contributing factor is a low value attached to this service (Chapter 3). Some women state quite directly that they did not think prenatal care was important or useful, some seem to fear it, some contend that other matters were more pressing than seeking out prenatal services, and some say care is important only if you feel sick. These personal perspectives have led the Committee to conclude that drawing more women into prenatal care will require increased public information and education about the nature and value of this care. This fourth goal supplements the three already noted: eliminating financial barriers, ensuring basic system capacity, and improving the organization and ambiance of services themselves.

● **We recommend that public and private groups—government, foundations, health services agencies, professional societies, and others—invest in a long-term, high-quality public information campaign to educate Americans about the importance of prenatal care for healthy mothers and infants and the need to begin such care early in pregnancy. The campaign should carry its message to schools, the media, family planning and other health care settings, social service networks, and places of employment. Additional campaigns should be aimed at the groups at highest risk for insufficient care. Whether directed at the entire population or a specific subgroup,** public information campaigns should always include specific instructions on where to go or whom to call to arrange for prenatal services.

We urge a serious effort to avoid one-shot, short-lived campaigns. Sporadic media flurries around such issues as low birthweight have been frequent in recent years, but few have been long-term and many have already fizzled without, we suspect, much impact on attitudes or behavior. We also underscore the importance of campaigns aimed at the groups that most often secure insufficient prenatal care, such as very young teenagers, low-income multiparous teenagers, uninsured women, women over 35 with several children, recent immigrants, certain high-risk minority groups, and very low-income women in both rural and inner-city areas (Chapters 1 and 2). Those who plan and implement campaigns to reach these groups should study in advance where the targeted individuals live, work, study, and play, and what they read, watch, and listen to. They must address their messages not only to pregnant women, but also to their male partners and their families. They must be aware of linguistic barriers and cultural influences. Put another way, audience definition, market research, premarket testing, and other skills of the advertising and marketing fields need to be applied to public education about prenatal care.

In addition to general information about what prenatal care is and why it is important, public information campaigns should include three themes: first, prenatal care is important even if a pregnant woman feels well; second, although previous pregnancies have been uneventful, subsequent ones may not be, and health supervision is important from early pregnancy on. Third, the signs and symptoms of pregnancy should be clearly explained. In addition to these messages about prenatal care and pregnancy, public information and education should emphasize basic concepts of family planning, given the strong association between whether a pregnancy is planned and onset of prenatal care (Chapter 2).

Schools especially should help in conveying such information. Although the topics of prenatal care and family planning are discussed in some health education programs, not all schools offer such education, and anecdotal information suggests that the quality of some health education is poor. Clearly, young people need to understand what prenatal care and family planning are and their importance in reproduction. Schools are in an excellent position to reach this population with high-quality education on these important topics.

Similarly, it is important that the health education offered as part of family planning services—both through groups and one-on-one counseling—include material on the importance of prenatal care. Because virtually all users of contraception are sexually active, it is highly appropriate that future pregnancies be discussed during visits to obtain contraception, even if avoidance of pregnancy is the main focus at the time. Such preconception counseling should cover the value of planning for pregnancy, the role of prenatal care in healthy birth outcomes, and how to obtain such care. When a woman enters the family planning system because she wishes a pregnancy test, additional opportunities for providing education about prenatal care arise. And, of course, if the test is positive and the woman elects to continue the pregnancy, she needs prompt referral for prenatal care and education to help her understand the importance of such care. This import referral opportunity—often missed—is discussed in more detail later.

Finally, we wish to underscore the simple notion that prenatal services must be advertised to prospective clients. New or existing services that no one knows about are not really accessible. Thus, public information campaigns about the importance of prenatal care—whether directed toward the general population or toward specific groups—should always explain how to arrange for care in a given community or through a specific program. This suggestion was made above in relation to the Medicaid program, but it applies equally to all programs that are attempting to serve women who are at risk for inadequate prenatal care.

THE ROLE OF OUTREACH: A GENERAL FRAMEWORK

Available data suggest that the four-part comprehensive program just outlined would lead to major improvements in the use of prenatal care. It would not bring about universal participation in prenatal care, however. The data presented in Chapters 1 through 3 suggest clearly that a variety of women will remain outside the system, despite major improvements, because of extreme social isolation or youth; apathy, fear, or denial; drug addiction; homelessness; fear of deportation, arrest, or other sanction; culturally based avoidance; and other concerns.

Figure 5.1 illustrates this point. Group A is the set of women who—because of adequate insurance, a well-functioning health care system in their community, personal resourcefulness, or all three—secure sufficient care. Group B is the set of women who would be able to obtain more adequate care were the four basic system changes made. The precise size of group B, of course, is unknown; however, data and program experience presented throughout this report suggest that it is substantial. The European data and experience summarized by Miller (see his paper at the end of this volume) show that rates of participation in prenatal care are high when the maternity system includes few barriers to care.

Group C is the residual, hard-to-reach population that would remain without prenatal care even after major system reforms had been made. As

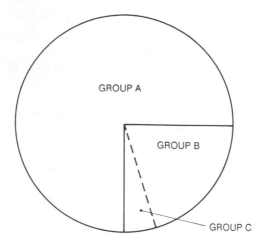

FIGURE 5.1   Proportion of pregnant women obtaining sufficient prenatal care under various organizational and financial arrangements.

with group B, the precise size of group C is unknown; it is probably small. For these women, special services are needed to locate and enroll them in prenatal care and then to provide them with enough support, attention, and caring that they do not drop out along the way. These two functions—casefinding and social support—are the activities defined in this report as outreach. In the two sections that follow, we offer some suggestions about how these services can be used to increase use of prenatal care among those who are hardest to reach.

Before doing so, however, we must stress our view that, at present, outreach services are being unfairly saddled with the burden of removing obstacles to prenatal care. Time and again, the Committee learned of communities that have invested in outreach to overcome basic inadequacies in existing networks of prenatal services, rather than changing the system itself. Faced with significant financial barriers, limited service capacity, inhospitable institutional practices, and a basic lack of public understanding about prenatal care, the response is often to hire outreach workers, or organize brief campaigns of posters in buses touting the importance of prenatal services, or arrange for compensatory social support rather than take on the more challenging task of repairing fundamental flaws. Repeatedly, outreach is organized to help women over and around major obstacles to care, but the obstacles themselves remain. The Committee gradually came to the conclusion that organizations whose primary focus is casefinding and social support seem, in the words of one member, to be "waging guerilla warfare" against institutions that are turning away patients, either deliberately or as an inadvertent consequence of their financial and other policies. Given that outreach programs typically have neither the resources nor the authority to bring about significant improvements in access to care, it is not surprising that their impact, though sometimes positive, is often limited (Chapter 4). Accordingly:

• We recommend that initiatives to increase use of prenatal care not rely on casefinding and social support to correct the major financial and institutional barriers that currently impede access. Rather, outreach should be only one component of a well-designed, well-functioning system and should be targeted toward women who remain unserved despite easily accessible services. Outreach should only be funded when it is linked to a highly accessible system of prenatal services, or, at a minimum, when it is part of a comprehensive plan to strengthen the system, emphasizing the four areas previously described.

To fund outreach in isolation and hope that, alone, it will lead to major improvements in the use of prenatal services is naive and wasteful.

CASEFINDING

Stressing again that outreach must be linked to improved—or improving—prenatal care systems, the Committee tried to learn which casefinding methods are most effective. Unfortunately, data assembled from the 31 programs studied were not sufficient to support clear recommendations about what techniques are indisputably the most useful. This weak science base is traceable primarily to difficulties in isolating the impact of a single casefinding method (usually, several are in place simultaneously) and the fact that data on casefinding efficacy are usually confounded by other aspects of the maternity care system. In addition, little research of any kind has been done in this area, probably because of the methodological problems just noted and because of its low status among health services researchers. What the Committee could distill about useful forms of casefinding is presented in Chapter 4. Based on the experiences summarized there and in Appendix A:

• We recommend that *in communities where financial and institutional barriers have been removed, or as part of a comprehensive plan to do so,* at least five kinds of casefinding be considered for their compatibility with a program's goals and constraints:

1. telephone hotline and referral services that can make prenatal appointments during the initial call and can provide assistance to callers in arranging needed maternity, health and social services;

2. television and, in particular, radio spots to announce specific services, coordinated with posters displayed in the mass transit system;

3. efforts to encourage current program participants to recruit additional participants from their friends, neighbors, and relatives;

4. strong referral ties between the prenatal program and a variety of other systems in which pregnant women at risk for insufficient care may be found: family planning clinics, schools, housing programs, WIC agencies, welfare and unemployment offices, churches and community service groups, shelters for the homeless, the police and corrections systems, substance-abuse programs and treatment centers, and other health and social service networks; and

5. outreach workers who work in carefully defined target areas and seek clients among well-defined target populations.

Whatever the method used, casefinding should be directed toward high-risk groups and areas. This requires that program leaders pinpoint the sociodemographic characteristics and geographic locations of women who obtain insufficient prenatal care.

The materials in Chapter 1 can help to define target groups, although the data discussed there are primarily national—states and communities need more detailed information on their own populations. Chapter 2 also presents information that can help to define target groups. Data from both chapters suggest that several populations are likely candidates for targeted casefinding (as they are for focused campaigns of public information): very young teenagers, low-income multiparous teenagers, women over 35 with several children, substance-abusing women and homeless women, recent immigrants, certain high-risk minority groups, and very low-income women in both inner-city and rural areas.

The fifth method highlighted above, use of outreach workers, requires comment. Much of the program data assembled by the Committee suggest that the effectiveness of these workers is limited. We suspect, though, that when such workers are used only in a carefully targeted way—in very low-income housing projects, for example, or other areas with high concentrations of women at risk for inadequate prenatal care, their effectiveness may be greater than some of the program data suggest. The personal touch they offer to women whose lives are often in chaos may be just what is needed, and the poorest inner cities and rural areas of America may need more of them. We emphasize again, though, the importance of their work being focused on areas of greatest need only, given the expense, labor-intensity, and occasional dangers of the job.

A final note on outreach workers. It is not uncommon for communities to have outreach workers from several different agencies working in a single area. Representatives from child abuse and neglect services, pediatrics, social services, sanitation, housing, and rat and poison control can all be knocking on the same doors. The potential for fear, suspicion, and lack of efficiency that such a scenario suggests leads us to a simple suggestion:

We recommend that communities experiment with multipurpose outreach workers in an effort to increase efficiency, enhance the receptivity of neighborhood residents, and, perhaps, increase the effectiveness of such workers. Evaluation should accompany well-designed trials of this approach and, if they are found useful, results should be widely disseminated.

We recognize a historical cycle here. Over the years, single-purpose and multipurpose outreach move in and out of style. In the early days of the War on Poverty, for example, the multiservice model was ascendant; in the 1980s it is rare. Our sense is that the pendulum has swung too far in the single-purpose direction and that a change is in order.

The Committee also calls particular attention to casefinding through closer links between pregnancy testing and prenatal services. A major opportunity to enroll pregnant women in prenatal care promptly is missed each time a positive pregnancy test is not accompanied by an appointment for prenatal services, if appropriate. Similarly, a negative pregnancy test signals that referral to family planning or even infertility services may be in order.

We recommend that pregnancy-testing services and prenatal care programs develop stronger referral ties, including the ability to make appointments for prenatal care at the pregnancy testing site. Missed prenatal appointments require vigorous follow-up.

In this context, we also urge that, given teenagers' poor use of prenatal care (especially teenagers who already have one or more children), schools include the availability of pregnancy testing in their health services and make special efforts to help pregnant teenagers obtain prenatal care. Health clinics based in schools are increasingly common and provide a natural setting for this function.

Similarly, pediatricians, family practitioners, and others caring for families with young children can help in the task of casefinding. In Chapter 1, the strong association between higher birth order and poor use of prenatal care was noted; young, poor, multiparous women in particular form an exceedingly high-risk group. This finding supports an additional suggestion:

We recommend that health care providers in touch with women who have young children—particularly low-income teenagers with young children— periodically raise the topics of family planning and child spacing. If additional children are planned or already on the way, the topic of prenatal care should be raised. Specific information on where and how to obtain prenatal care should be easily available in these settings.

We also urge that careful thought be given to the mechanics of linking prenatal services more directly to pregnancy testing and pediatric services. In particular, referral systems must ensure that patient confidentiality and sensitivity are respected. To help develop and disseminate information about this method of casefinding, it would be useful to describe and evaluate alternative approaches.

On a more general level, we also emphasize that casefinding—by whatever method—can be time-consuming, expensive, and difficult to conduct. For example, high-risk groups who remain outside the maternity care system may resist efforts to draw them into care and be difficult to engage; casefinding through outreach workers requires a significant investment in recruitment, training, support, and supervision; developing appealing placards for subways and buses often requires careful graphic design, market research and premarket-testing, and extensive negotiations with local transit authorities. Yet it is our impression that in planning and raising funds for prenatal care programs, the casefinding function is often shortchanged.

We recommend that those responsible for planning and funding prenatal programs recognize explicitly that casefinding is not simple and may be costly. Program planning and budgeting should provide adequate, realistic support for casefinding.

SOCIAL SUPPORT

Ample data show that with the care and attention of a single person or two (a patient advocate, a case manager, a granny, or whatever), high-risk women can be helped to obtain adequate prenatal care and to secure the many ancillary services they need (see Appendix A).

Were the four recommendations for improving the maternity system implemented, the need for social support might decrease, because women would not need as much help arranging for care. Even in a well-functioning system of prenatal services, however, Group C (see Figure 5.1) would remain, requiring concentrated support and assistance. Accordingly:

• **We recommend that programs providing prenatal services to high-risk, often low-income groups include social support services to help maintain participation in care and arrange for additional services as needed. Home visiting is an important form of social support and should be available in programs caring for high-risk women.**

Sometimes the primary obstetric care provider fills this social support role; sometimes the task is delegated to others. Whatever the arrangement, this function needs to be adequately financed (and, in particular, reimbursed through public and private insurance), as it, like casefinding, can be time-consuming and therefore expensive.

However, having made this general point, we are reluctant to urge that "case management," as it is currently being used in the administration of the Medicaid program, be widely applied. As a recent survey of state Medicaid directors noted, "Case management lacks a precise conceptual or operational definition. In the absence of a definition, case management typically describes a range of activities that can vary from routine, minimally professional referral services, to primary nursing, to comprehensive care plan development, oversight, and monitoring."[8] This situation leads to an additional suggestion:

We recommend that the federal government, in partnership with states, providers, consumers, and public and private insurers, develop clear standards and performance criteria for the function of case management. These standards and criteria must be unequivocally oriented toward women's health and social needs. Once developed, they should be adopted in a wide range of prenatal settings, particularly those caring for significant numbers of high-risk women, and all payment systems should support such care.

In concluding these sections on casefinding and social support, the Committee again stresses that they do not substitute for the basic system repairs outlined earlier. Program leaders and policymakers concerned with increasing use of prenatal care should concentrate first and foremost on financial and institutional issues and should not be seduced into thinking that more limited measures such as hotlines or outreach workers will solve the problem. Instituting an outreach program may appear less difficult and expensive than fundamental system reform; it may also have considerable public relations value. But the Committee strongly suggests that outreach should be aimed only at carefully defined high-risk groups and that it should be an adjunct to a well-functioning system that is easily accessible to the vast majority of pregnant women.

MANAGEMENT AND EVALUATION

The Committee's study of programs yielded several observations about management and evaluation (Chapter 4). On the basis of these findings:

● **We recommend that programs to improve participation in prenatal care invest generously in planning and assessment of needs. Doing so will require a deeper appreciation, among funders in particular, of the** time needed for responsible, intelligent program design and planning. Substantial improvements in the use of prenatal care (or in other measures of outcome such as low birthweight or infant mortality) should not be expected too soon.

Issues to be considered in basic planning and needs assessment include in-depth reviews of existing maternity services, provider practices, and attitudes; public and private health insurance coverage in the target state or community; the views of local women regarding existing maternity services; careful definition of the target populations, of local barriers to prenatal care, of existing community services, and of relevant historical and political realities; market research and premarket testing of materials (where applicable); design and testing of management information systems or other mechanisms for providing basic program data (who is being served, how staff and other resources are being used, program changes over time, and so on); and consideration of whether a formal evaluation should be included, and, if so, what type.

Far too many of the programs reviewed by the Committee were deficient in conducting these basic functions, even programs receiving public funds and in existence for many years. Many programs came into existence quite quickly—often because of the sudden availability of money or opportunity—and were in business before a number of important preliminary steps could be taken. Funders, policymakers, and particularly politicians need to understand that these programs—like human services generally—cannot be organized in a hurried, slipshod manner; information needed for planning takes time to gather and analyze.

The Committee noted a reluctance to view investments in prenatal care programs as long-term commitments whose impact should not be anticipated too soon. Developing new statewide networks of clinics, changing community views about the value of a service such as prenatal care, encouraging more private physicians to care for low-income patients, convincing a community that a certain care facility is now receptive to immigrant women, or developing trust in a particular community worker are all difficult tasks that take generous amounts of time. We were distressed by the number of programs that felt under pressure to show "results" (such as a dramatic increase in first-trimester enrollment in prenatal care or a marked decrease in low birthweight) in a year or so, sometimes less. Common sense alone suggests that many of the types of programs outlined in the Appendix take several years to develop into smoothly functioning services and sometimes longer to show results, if any. Moreover, no single approach (such as a media campaign or a modest expansion in Medicaid eligibility) should be under pressure to correct such complicated problems as infant mortality or low birthweight.

With regard to program evaluation:

• **We recommend that early in a program's course its directors decide whether it is to be primarily a service program (with data collected mainly to help in program development and monitoring) or whether it is also to test an idea in the field. The latter type requires ample funding if the evaluation is to be sound; it also requires sophisticated systems for data collection and experts in program evaluation—resources that must be built into the program from the outset.**

This recommendation carries the implicit message that although all programs should be carefully managed, not all should be evaluated. Meaningful evaluation is often expensive, drawing resources from other activities that may be more urgent; moreover, it requires control or comparison groups, which many operating programs cannot establish. It requires significant technical skill and expertise, as well as adequate investments in research design, computer software, and data entry and analysis.

For programs that choose to include a strong evaluation component, specific consideration should be given to qualitative versus quantitative approaches and to the possibility of randomized trials and alternative designs that attempt to overcome selection bias. We also note that a higher quality of effort is needed than that exhibited by most of the programs reviewed. Indeed, the Committee found that significant amounts of time and money are being wasted on evaluation studies that are so flawed methodologically as to be almost useless.

RESEARCH

The Committee found a number of topics that merit research. Before listing them, however, we assert that no further research should be conducted to show the importance of financial and institutional barriers in the poor use of prenatal care. More than enough data documenting these relationships exist, even if public policy addressing these problems is inadequate. We do urge, however, that any community designing programs to increase early use of prenatal care carefully assess the *extent* of financial barriers, inadequate system capacity, and inhospitable institutional practices. For example, in many communities only anecdotal information exists regarding the availability of prenatal services: whether certain clinics are overloaded, and if so, to what extent; the fees at area clinics; and so forth. Obtaining such basic information should be the first order of business in designing prenatal programs..

We are reluctant to recommend extensive research on the relative effectiveness of various casefinding activities, i.e., assessing the client-yield of community workers versus hotlines or financial incentives. These activities are usually so intertwined with other variables in the system that methodologically sound studies of their impact would be virtually impossible to design. Moreover, given the major role that financial and institutional barriers play in determining use of prenatal care, it seems almost diversionary to study outreach techniques rather than to improve the basic prenatal care system. With this context in mind:

● We recommend that *in communities where financial and institutional obstacles to care have been significantly lowered,* research be undertaken on several topics:

1. Why do some pregnant women register late—or not at all—for prenatal care even when financial and institutional barriers are ostensibly absent? In particular, what are the emotional and attitudinal factors that limit participation in care?

2. How can the content of prenatal care be revised to encourage women to seek such care early in pregnancy?

3. What casefinding techniques are most helpful in identifying very high-risk groups (such as low-income multiparous teenagers) and linking them to prenatal services?

4. What are the costs associated with various forms of casefinding and social support?

5. What are the most effective ways to forge links between physicians in private practice and community agencies providing the ancillary health and social services that high-risk women often need?

6. How is access to maternity services being affected by such recent developments as the decreased ability of hospitals to finance care for indigent patients through cost-shifting, the increase in corporate ownership of hospitals, the gradual expansion of the DRG (diagnosis-related groups) system beyond the Medicare program, and the increasing profit orientation of the health care sector generally?

With regard to the first topic, it would be helpful if researchers could use similar theoretical frameworks and lists of barriers when interviewing women. As Chapter 3 shows, many questionnaires have been developed, but their diversity hampers efforts to synthesize findings. One particular issue that research of this type might probe is why some women who are clearly pleased to be pregnant seek pregnancy confirmation early but then do not arrange for prenatal care, even in areas where the maternity care system is functioning well.

The second topic suggests that early enrollment in prenatal services might increase if such care were more clearly directed to major issues in the first trimester of pregnancy. These include: the steps women can take to protect the health and development of the fetus (such as avoiding x-rays, alcohol and other drugs); the discomforts of early pregnancy (such as nausea, worries about "getting fat," and changing personal relationships occasioned by the pregnancy); and the ambivalence or negative feelings that some women experience when first learning they are pregnant. If prenatal care gave more emphasis to these first trimester issues, and if women better understood that prenatal care was helpful and important from conception onward, use of this health service might well increase.

The third topic should include such questions as: (1) What is the relative effectiveness of such case-finding techniques as community canvassing via outreach workers, telephone canvassing, hotlines, public service announcements, and/or provision of various incentives? Do some approaches work better in some settings and for some target groups? (2) How can referral links between prenatal care and other services in which high-risk women participate best be developed and maintained? (3) What institutional homes (health departments, social services agencies, freestanding institutions) are best suited to various outreach activities?

The fourth topic—costs—merits emphasis. With very few exceptions— the Central Harlem Outreach Program of New York City being the shining example—the programs reviewed by the Committee had little or no data linking program costs to client outcomes. To compete for future support and to provide more accountability, such data need to be collected.

The fifth topic addresses the problem of private practitioners being isolated from many community-based agencies that provide the supplementary services some of their patients need, such as WIC and substance abuse treatment. Research in this area should proceed with the full involvement of private practitioners so that conclusions will be acceptable to them and relevant to their practices.

Our sixth and final suggestion for research simply acknowledges that fact that current changes in the health care system may be decreasing access to prenatal care. If so, such influences need to be carefully described and quantified, and policymakers should be alerted to the findings of such investigations.

A NOTE TO FUNDERS

We conclude with some observations directed to those who fund prenatal services: public agencies, legislative bodies, and private foundations and voluntary groups. Many of these points have been covered elsewhere under various headings. We collect and reiterate them here for emphasis.

Over the years, private and public institutions have funded a variety of demonstration and research programs in the general area of prenatal care for low-income groups. The Committee has reviewed many of these programs and has concluded that at least three problems cloud the relationship between these programs and their sponsors.

First, the absence of reliable and consistent funding of prenatal care programs for low-income groups often forces program directors to ask foundations or government for research and demonstration funds that in fact are used—out of necessity—to subsidize basic program services. It is for this reason, perhaps, that the Committee found very little real innovation or research in the areas of delivery of prenatal care or outreach for low-income groups. In the Committee's view, fostering high-quality research on complicated issues of access to care will require government, foundations, and program directors to give up the fiction of subsidizing direct services through research grants.

Second, the Committee found that many research and demonstration programs are funded by foundations and government for 2 or 3 years. These short funding cycles have at least two negative consequences. First, they require program leaders to spend large amounts of time searching for funds, responding rapidly to competitive grant announcements, preparing numerous funding applications, lobbying state legislatures and other public groups for support, and so on. Coupled with often burdensome reporting requirements, the struggle to maintain funding has become debilitating and frustrating. Second, the short cycles carry the implicit message that programs must implement, evaluate, and show results within 2 or 3 years. Program directors are aware that their funding may depend upon their ability to provide these results quickly. Such a process suggests a lack of understanding of the basic facts of organizational sociology. To implement and institutionalize change in any organization or client population requires considerable time. The Committee suggests that genuine innovation and evaluation cannot be accomplished in much less than 5 years and that to expect valid results in less time is naive.

Third, although both government and foundations have regularly funded demonstration projects in the area of prenatal care for poor women, often with considerable public fanfare, support of successful programs over many years is less evident. The Committee suggests that foundations and government might more usefully serve this area of health care by working together, in a deliberate and planned fashion, to ensure that programs whose value and effectiveness have been proven are maintained "when the grant runs out." A conscious plan for moving innovation into the mainstream would allow those responsible for health care to use their energies in more constructive and innovative ways. It would also enable useful programs to continue when the next social priority comes along claiming attention and funds.

SUMMARY

In the long run, the best prospects for improving use of prenatal care—and reversing current declines—lie in reorganizing the nation's maternity care system. Although a new system may include some elements of the existing one, the Committee specifically recommends against the current practice of making incremental changes in programs already in place; instead it argues for fundamental reform. Several ways are available for designing the specific components of a new system, but no such work should proceed until the nation's leaders first make a commitment to enact substantial changes. A deeper commitment to family planning services and education should accompany improvements in the maternity care system.

In the short term, we urge strengthening existing systems through which women secure prenatal services. This includes simultaneous actions to remove financial barriers to care, make certain that basic system capacity is adequate for all women, improve the policies and practices that shape prenatal services at the delivery site, and increase public information and education about prenatal care. Federal leadership of this four-part program is essential, supplemented by state action to ensure the availability of prenatal services to all residents.

Even if all four system changes were implemented, there would still be some women without sufficient care because of extreme social isolation, youth, fear or denial, drug addiction, cultural factors, or other reasons. For these women, there is a clear need for casefinding and social support to locate and enroll them in prenatal services and to encourage continuation in care once it is begun. These outreach services, built onto a well-designed, highly accessible system of prenatal services, can help draw the most hard-to-reach women into care.

Unfortunately, though, outreach is often undertaken without first making certain that the basic maternity care system is accessible and responsive to women's needs. Too often, communities organize outreach to help women over and around major obstacles to care rather than removing the obstacles themselves. Thus, the Committee specifically urges that outreach be funded only when linked to a well-functioning system of prenatal services or, at a minimum, when it is part of a comprehensive plan that emphasizes four areas noted above. To fund outreach in isolation and hope that it alone will accomplish major improvements in the use of prenatal services is naive and wasteful.

In support of this general view, the Committee also makes a number of recommendations regarding program management, evaluation, and research. The Committee concludes that not all programs should have to muster the funds and expertise to conduct meaningful evaluation. For those that choose to do so, a higher quality of effort is needed than that exhibited by most of the programs reviewed. With regard to research, the Committee specifically urges that no more research be conducted to demonstrate the importance of financial and other institutional barriers to care. We do, however, suggest six specific research topics and recommend that the current practice of securing funds for services under the guise of research cease.

REFERENCES AND NOTES

1. Select Panel for the Promotion of Health. Better Health for Our Children: A National Strategy, Vol. 1. DHHS Pub. No. (PHS) 79-55071. Washington, D.C.: Government Printing Office, 1981.
2. American College of Obstetricians and Gynecologists. Standards of Obstetric-Gynecologic Services, 6th ed. Washington, D.C., 1985.
3. American Academy of Pediatrics and American College of Obstetricians and Gynecologists. Guidelines for Perinatal Care. Washington, D.C., 1983.
4. A final report of the Expert Panel on the Content of Prenatal Care is expected early in 1989.
5. The Institute of Medicine has a study under way at present on the effects of medical liability on the delivery of maternal and child health care. A final report is expected in early 1989.
6. American Hospital Association. Medicaid Options: State Opportunities and Strategies for Expanding Eligibility. Chicago, 1987.
7. Additional observations on private sector leadership in improving insurance coverage for maternity services are in National Commission to Prevent Infant Mortality. The Private Sector's Role in Reducing Infant Mortality. Washington, D.C., 1988.
8. Luehrs J. Issue Brief: Case Management as an Optional Medicaid Service. Washington, D.C.: Health Policy Studies, National Governors' Association, September 1986, p. 3.

Summaries of the 31 Programs Studied

To identify programs that might provide data on increasing and sustaining adequate use of prenatal care, the Committee and staff:

- reviewed survey data assembled in Spring 1985 by the national Healthy Mothers/Healthy Babies coalition;
- sent letters in August 1986 and March 1987 to all directors of state maternal and child health agencies, requesting assistance in identifying data on the relative effectiveness of various outreach activities in their states;
- contacted organizations active in maternal and child health, including advocacy groups (such as the Children's Defense Fund), foundations (such as the Ford Foundation), and professional societies (such as the American College of Obstetricians and Gynecologists);
- queried other organizations known to be conducting research in prenatal care, including the Alan Guttmacher Institute, the Office of Technology Assessment, the American Hospital Association, the Centers for Disease Control, and the General Accounting Office;
- commissioned an update of the report on statewide prenatal care initiatives issued in 1986 by the Center for Population and Family Health, Columbia University School of Public Health;
- commissioned a paper reviewing comprehensive service programs for pregnant teenagers funded by the Office of Adolescent Family Life Programs within the U.S. Department of Health and Human Services;
- ran an advertisement in *The Nation's Health* (newspaper of the American Public Health Association) requesting program leads; and

• discussed the project with members of the public health and medical care communities, and reviewed journals and reports in which relevant material might be published.

From these sources, a master list of almost 200 programs was compiled. Each program was contacted directly by telephone or mail or both to learn more about its activities and to ascertain whether it had adequate data to judge its effectiveness in improving participation in prenatal care. Written reports from projects were reviewed, and in some instances program directors were asked to work with Committee staff to develop summaries of programmatic activities and data. Out of these approximately 200 programs, 31 were selected for more intensive study and are described in this appendix. The criteria used in the selection process are discussed in Chapter 4.

An important part of the program review was a workshop held in May 1987 during which the Committee talked in depth with the leaders of eight programs using varied means of improving use of prenatal care. These informal conversations provided valuable insight into the history and context of these and other programs.

Program directors, particularly directors of projects not already described in the published literature, were closely involved in drafting the summaries that follow. They emphasize each program's origins, its principal activities, and evidence that it has influenced registration or continuation in prenatal care. Most note the year of each program's initiation, key factors in its inception, funding sources, and whether the program is still under way. Unfortunately, very few projects were able to supply the committee with data on program costs in relation to impact (that is, cost-benefit data of some type); consequently, most of the summaries do not include such information. As will be evident, the program descriptions vary in length, depth, and intensity of data. This reflects the diversity of the programs, wide variations in their ability to provide clear descriptions of their activities, and differences in the amount of relevant information they could supply.

Chapter 4 describes the five categories developed by the Committee to group the many programs reviewed briefly and the 31 studied in detail. As noted there, programs were classified on the basis of their major emphasis.

TYPE 1: PROGRAMS TO REDUCE FINANCIAL BARRIERS

The Committee studied two programs that take a direct approach to reducing financial barriers to care: the Healthy Start Program in Massachusetts and the Prenatal–Postpartum Care Program in Michigan.

Healthy Start Program—Massachusetts[1]

Massachusetts initiated its Healthy Start Program in December 1985. The genesis of the program was similar to that of many others reviewed by the Committee: a rise in infant mortality rates followed by the appointment of a Blue Ribbon Task Force and implementation of at least some of the Task Force's recommendations. The scope of the Massachusetts program, however, is broader than that of many of the other programs reviewed. Most programs start small, involving a limited number of providers, one city, or a few counties. The Massachusetts program started statewide and was designed to include all willing providers. Healthy Start, a joint effort of the state health and welfare departments, offers financing for a full range of maternity services for any pregnant woman who lives in Massachusetts, is not currently enrolled in Medicaid, has no private health insurance, and has a family income at or below 200 percent (originally, 185 percent) of the federally defined poverty level.* Healthy Start funds can also be used to underwrite the initial care of women who are potentially eligible for Medicaid. Once such a woman has begun prenatal care through the Healthy Start program, her financial status is reviewed carefully; if she is found to be Medicaid-eligible in fact, that financing source (rather than Healthy Start) eventually covers her prenatal care costs.

The program is noteworthy for emphasizing expansion of the range of sites, including private providers, where low-income women can receive services, rather than taking the usual route of enlarging the capacity of existing settings where low-income women have traditionally received care. A pregnant woman enrolled in Healthy Start decides where she wishes to receive care, and as long as that provider is enrolled in the program, she may receive care there. Healthy Start staff believe that the program's focus on freedom of choice is one of its most important elements. Women who cannot or do not want to travel long distances, who have a good relationship with a current provider, or who do not want to use a particular facility have no reason to delay seeking care, because they can make the arrangements they prefer, provided that their chosen caregiver participates in the program.

After completing a very simple registration process, all obstetrician–gynecologists, family practitioners, pediatricians, medical specialists and other health care providers, health centers, hospitals, laboratories, and

---

*As this report is being written, Massachusetts has raised its Medicaid income eligibility ceiling to 185 percent of the federal poverty level. This expansion will result in about 80 percent of Healthy Start clients being transferred to the Medicaid program. The state has also passed landmark legislation that significantly expands the availability of health insurance to all state residents.

pharmacies are eligible for reimbursement for services provided to Healthy Start participants. The registration procedure is intentionally less cumbersome than that required to become certified as a Medicaid provider. Registration has also been made easy for the woman. She may apply through her care provider or by calling a statewide toll-free number (1-800-531-BABY). The application form can be completed at home and mailed in, thus avoiding any "welfare taint" that can accompany applying for Medicaid.

Healthy Start covers all "medical care necessary to maintain health during pregnancy" plus one pediatric visit. Although the program does not require a particular type or "package" of care, women who call the project's 800 number for a referral are sent, when possible, to comprehensive services in their communities. Healthy Start originally reimbursed for hospital labor and delivery costs as well, but these expenses have recently been shifted to the Hospital Free Care Pool. Providers are reimbursed at the Medicaid rate for physicians and community health centers and at the non-Medicaid Public Assistance Rate for hospitals. The average cost per program participant has been $1,100 for prenatal care and $2,200 for hospitalization. The estimated cost of Healthy Start in the 1987 fiscal year was $20.3 million.

A preliminary evaluation of Healthy Start has been conducted using program records, hospital discharge data, birth certificates, focus group discussions, and informal interviews with program staff.[2] One major finding is that the program has been successful in enrolling providers. As of February 1988, all hospital-based prenatal clinics, all health centers with prenatal care services, and more than 2,000 physicians and nurse–midwives, including 476 obstetricians (some of whom were not certified as Medicaid providers) had agreed to serve Healthy Start clients. The program enrolled 65 percent of all uninsured pregnant women and estimates that it enrolled 85 percent of the women eligible for the program on the basis of income. Forty percent of Healthy Start participants used private providers. The program's penetration has been particularly high among minorities, teenagers, the unmarried, and those with less than a high school education.

Another major component of the evaluation is a comparison between Healthy Start participants and those insured under other programs or uninsured. Covering the period of July through December 1986, this analysis was made possible by the inclusion on Massachusetts birth certificates of source of payment for prenatal care. More than 40,000 birth certificates were analyzed and over 2,000 were of babies born to Healthy Start participants. In general, the evaluation showed that Healthy Start was more successful in helping women to maintain participation in care once begun than to initiate care early. Controlling for demographic differences in the composition of the various groups defined by payor status, Healthy Start participants were found to be more likely than those on Medicaid to initiate care in the first 4 months of pregnancy, but less likely to do so than those with private or other government insurance or the uninsured. Participants were also found more likely than all groups except those with private insurance or whose insurance status was unknown to have utilized care adequately, defined as 80 percent or more of the visits recommended by the American College of Obstetricians and Gynecologists (see Chapter 1), adjusted for the timing of initiation of care. The largest difference in rates of remaining in care was among the highest risk groups: blacks, teenagers, and the unmarried. These differences, suggesting that Healthy Start participants received more quantitatively adequate prenatal care, are supported by comparisons of pregnancy outcomes (low birthweight and prematurity) across payor groups, which also show Healthy Start having a positive impact. The evaluators attribute the the program's success in improving pregnancy outcomes to its emphasis on enhancing the continuity and content of care, greater participation among program enrollees in programs such as WIC, and decreased maternal strain because the program reduces worries about paying for maternity care.

Prenatal–Postpartum Care Program—Michigan[3]

In 1981, Michigan recorded an increase in its rate of infant mortality, a development that many experts in the state linked to the recession during the early 1980s and the resultant loss of health insurance by many families and individuals. To address this increase, the governor established a Director's Special Task Force on Prenatal Care. In 1984, this group released its findings and recommendations in *Prenatal Care: A Healthy Beginning for Michigan's Children*. The major recommendation of the report was that the state establish a program to finance prenatal care for women who were ineligible for Medicaid and had no private health insurance—that is, the uninsured, many of whom worked in jobs that provided no health insurance or were married to men who had lost their jobs or health insurance during the recession.

Receptive to this recommendation, the state legislature passed a bill in 1984 that established the Prenatal–Postpartum Care (PPC) Program and in 1986 declared prenatal and postpartum care a "basic health service" in state law. As such, these services are to be made available and accessible to all state residents in need of the services without regard for place of residence, marital status, sex, age, race, or inability to pay. In fiscal year (FY) 1984–1985, about $2.5 million was allocated to begin phasing in the PPC program; for FY 1985–1986 and FY 1986–1987, $5 million dollars was provided. By 1988, the appropriation had grown to $5.9 million.

The program began enrolling clients around January 1, 1985. It covers women at or below 185 percent of the federal poverty level who are not enrolled in the Medicaid program. In addition, as in Massachusetts, funds may be used to underwrite the cost of early prenatal care for women who may become Medicaid recipients later in their pregnancies. Once Medicaid eligibility is established, Medicaid funds are used instead of PPC monies. Services covered include medical care during pregnancy (using ACOG standards) and one postpartum visit. Also included are outreach and referral to prenatal care, nutritional and psychosocial assessments, vitamins, routine laboratory procedures, patient education, and referral for high-risk prenatal services; limited reimbursement is available for special tests, procedures, and medications. It is important to note that the PPC program primarily reimburses for a basic package of low-risk services. Women at high risk of poor pregnancy outcomes require additional nursing, nutrition, and social work services. These ancillary services have historically been available in some geographic areas through the state health department's Maternity and Infant Care (MIC) Projects and its Infant Health Improvement Projects (IHIP). Health departments in these areas use PPC and either MIC or IHIP funds to provide a more comprehensive set of prenatal services. PPC does not guarantee availability of care in a woman's county of residence or by a woman's provider of choice; it does not pay for inpatient care, nor does it pay for most special services that a high-risk pregnancy might require. The program originally did not include payment to physicians for labor and delivery services; however, such payment was added January 1, 1988.

The PPC program is administered through the Michigan Department of Public Health and its 48 local health departments. Local health departments either contract with area providers [private physicians, hospital clinics, health maintenance organizations (HMOs) or others] or, less often, provide the services themselves. Participating prividers must agree to offer the specified services and to accept Medicaid patients (to ensure continuity of care for those PPC women who become eligible for Medicaid during the pregnancy). Providers are reimbursed on a global fee basis, now including labor and delivery services, as noted above.

During the first full program year, 1985, 32 of the state's local health departments adopted the PPC program. By October 1986, 47 had. It is not known how many providers statewide have contracted with these local departments to provide care or what proportion were private physicians, hospital clinics, HMOs, or others. However, a recent survey conducted by a regional arm of the Michigan Healthy Mothers, Healthy Babies Coalition found that in 27 counties composing roughly one-third of the state, 33 percent of all prenatal providers accept Medicaid patients, and 26 percent accept both Medicaid and PPC. Leaders of the PPC Program report that some local health departments have been very successful in drawing individual providers into the program; others have had more trouble, particularly in areas with a limited number of settings offering prenatal care. In these areas, local health departments have tried to enlarge basic system capacity or to develope alternative provider systems, such as nurse–midwifery clinics. In 1986 the state health department and state Medicaid agency gave funds to several local health departments to address problems in system capacity, particularly those caused by the growing liability crisis. These grants could be used either to underwrite a portion of the physician's liability premium for each PPC or Medicaid client served or to establish nurse–midwifery clinics in areas with few or no providers. One county established such a clinic. All local agencies reported that under-writing liability premiums helped keep providers participating in the program.

Data on the use of prenatal care by program enrollees are available for 1985 and 1986. In 1985 about 2,500 women participated in PPC; 47 percent began prenatal care in the first trimester of care and 18 percent began in the third. In 1986 enrollment grew to 6,000 women; 55 percent began care in the first trimester, and 10 percent began in the third. In 1987 enrollment grew to 8,350 women. Data are not yet available on this group's patterns of care.

Although there are no baseline data against which to evaluate these statistics, the program appears to have increased marginally the percentage of women seeking care early in pregnancy. Program leaders report that, between 1985 and 1986, many program procedures were smoothed and administrative problems eased. The program became better known among social service workers and health professionals generally. News of the program spread by word-of-mouth, and the various techniques used to publicize the program became more extensive and better organized (the baby showers program and the 961-BABY hotline, described later in this appendix, both included PPC as one of their referral listings). In particular, the number of local health departments participating in PPC increased significantly between 1985 and 1986.

Type 2: Programs to Increase System Capacity

Four programs were studied that improve use of prenatal care by expanding the capacity of the clinic systems relied on by low-income women for their prenatal care. The four are: the Obstetrical Access Pilot Project in 13 counties in California; the Perinatal Program in Lea County, New Mexico; the Prenatal Care Assistance Program in New York State; and the Prevention of Low Birthweight Program in Onondaga County, New

York. The first two in particular emphasized developing services for poor women where few had existed for this population before.

Obstetrical Access Pilot Project—California[4]

The Obstetrical Access Pilot Project (OB Access) was developed in the late 1970s in California to address the fact that, despite the enactment of Medi-Cal (the California Medicaid program), serious gaps existed in the availability and extent of perinatal services for low-income women, particularly in certain geographic areas and ethnic groups. The proportion of California obstetricians who accepted Medi-Cal patients actually declined from 65 percent in 1974 to 46 percent in 1977. Patients and communities complained that many low-income women, both those eligible for Medi-Cal and others were experiencing severe problems in finding physicians with formal training and experience in obstetrics. Also, an increasing number of physicians were complaining about their inability to provide adequate care at the prevailing Medi-Cal reimbursement rates. In 1977, an emergency statute was enacted to revise physician reimbursement and stimulate Medi-Cal provider participation in primary and maternity care. By 1979, however, it was clear that the initiative was not having the desired effects, and a formal legislative resolution was passed so stating.

In the wake of this incident, the OB Access Pilot Project emerged (1) to provide better access to comprehensive and early obstetric services for Medi-Cal eligible mothers in areas where there were no obstetricians or where providers declined to participate in Medi-Cal and (2) as a consequence of improving access, to reduce the incidence of low birthweight and the associated incidence of perinatal morbidity and mortality. OB Access was a pilot program to test the feasibility and impact of providing reimbursement for a comprehensive package of perinatal services under Medi-Cal. The project operated for 3 years (1979–1982) and registered almost 7,000 women.

OB Access' comprehensive care included psychosocial and nutritional assessments, perinatal education (health, labor, delivery, and parenting education), and an initial outpatient well-baby examination, in addition to routine antepartum, intrapartum, and postpartum care (11 recommended examinations), prenatal vitamins, and routine laboratory tests (generally blood and urine analyses). The assessments determined what, if any, psychosocial, nutritional, or educational risks were present; when problems were detected, counseling was provided and referrals to other services were made as needed. Formal birth education classes were also provided.

Following an application and review process, seven community clinics and four county health departments (one in collaboration with a university hospital) were selected as OB Access providers. These were located in obstetrically underserved areas and appeared to be able to provide the amount and range of services specified. All the sites used a variety of methods to inform pregnant women of their programs. These included public service announcements on radio and television, newspaper articles, informational brochures, community meetings, and the casefinding efforts of welfare workers. The evaluators commented, however, that "the most effective method appeared to be word-of-mouth from patients who were satisfied with the care that they were receiving."

A full-scale evaluation of OB Access was conducted. With regard to initiation of care, evaluators found in the OB Access counties a reduction in the weighted average percent of inadequate care among pregnancies terminating in a live birth, from 10.15 percent in 1978 to 5.49 percent in 1982, a 45.9 percent decrease. (Inadequate care was defined as care begun in the third trimester, no care, or unknown care.) During the same period in the entire state, the percentage with inadequate care dropped from 10.0 percent to 6.60 percent, a 34.0 percent decrease; the reasons for this statewide decrease have not been defined. A second analysis compared the percentage of OB Access participants who received care in the first trimester with a matched group of Medi-Cal women. The results were negative, that is, the percentage of women who began care in the first trimester was higher in the Medi-Cal group.

The evaluation also suggested that the project had reduced the rate of low birthweight among program participants, which in turn formed the basis for benefit-cost analyses. It was estimated that every new dollar spent on OB Access services would save between $1.70 and $2.60, principally through reduced expenditures for neonatal intensive care. These estimates did not include any additional state administrative costs or start-up costs.

The cost-effectiveness data in particular convinced the California legislature to extend the program. In 1984, a bill was passed establishing the Comprehensive Perinatal Services Program, which requires that OB Access services be made available to all pregnant women enrolled in Medi-Cal. A closely related program currently in operation is the Community-Based Perinatal Services (CBPS) Program, which provides comprehensive perinatal care (prenatal care in particular) to low-income women (that is, women whose incomes fall below 200 percent of the federal poverty level). In 1986, CBPS served about 30,000 women.

Perinatal Program—Lea County, New Mexico[5]

One of the programs funded under the Robert Wood Johnson Foundation's Rural Infant Care Program was in Lea County, New Mexico, a relatively wealthy county that nevertheless had an infant death rate in 1980 of 19.8, 80 percent higher than the state average and among the highest county rates in the nation.

Problems obtaining prenatal care, delivery services, and assistance with infants' medical problems were described in the application for funding prepared by the University of New Mexico School of Medicine (Department of Pediatrics). It was the horror story found only too often in underserved areas. Many physicians required patients to pay in advance for prenatal care, even if they had insurance. This meant that a woman had to find $600 to $800 before she was accepted for her first visit. The local health department provided no prenatal care, nor did its nurses make home visits. The local hospital was operated by a for-profit chain and had no outpatient prenatal clinics. The result of these limitations was that approximately 20 percent of the women who delivered in the local hospital were walk-ins, defined as women who came to the emergency room for delivery having had five or fewer prenatal visits or no prenatal care at all. Others chose to go to Texas for prenatal care or labor and delivery, or both, claiming that these services cost less and were more easily accessible there. A survey of barriers to prenatal care in Lea County showed that, among 92 women who had received little or no care during a recent pregnancy, financial barriers were the explanation most commonly given.

Foundation funding made it possible for the medical school, working with the community, to develop ways to reduce infant mortality and increase access to prenatal care. A proposal to have the local health department operate prenatal clinics was turned down by the local physicians. According to the physician who coordinated the foundation grant, the local physicians argued that a county as wealthy as theirs would have few medically indigent families. They believed that those women who did not receive adequate prenatal care probably lacked motivation or education or both, and that other factors not associated with financial need accounted for the poor enrollment in prenatal care. A health department clinic, therefore, might compete with the private sector, attracting women who could afford private care but chose instead to use a "government giveaway program." Furthermore, local physicians were adamantly opposed to having a nurse–practitioner or other nonphysician provide prenatal care, as some had suggested.

An alternative plan was suggested by the community physicians and implemented in December 1980. Two women were employed to identify pregnant women in need of prenatal care (casefinding), to provide transportation, translation, and follow-up services for the women and their infants, and to serve as community health educators. Potential program participants identified by these community workers were then interviewed by a community coordinator to establish financial eligibility, to identify medical and social issues that required referrals, and to function as a liaison among the various program components. More than half of the physicians with obstetrical privileges at the local hospital agreed to care for eligible women in their offices on a sliding fee schedule, or without charge, if necessary. Medically indigent women were assigned to these physicians on a rotating basis for both prenatal care and delivery. The health department did pregnancy testing and routine laboratory work and distributed prenatal vitamins and iron. The March of Dimes and the Levi Strauss Company provided funds for supplementary services and prescription drugs. Additional funding was also provided by the state's Crippled Children's Services agency to finance the program and to support program evaluation.

It soon became apparent to the private physicians in the area that the unmet need for prenatal care among indigent women was significant and beyond their capacity or willingness to accommodate. It was not uncommon, for example, for women referred to private physicians by the community coordinator to report a 3- to 4-month waiting time for a first prenatal appointment, because the private physicians limited the number of indigent patients they would accommodate. Accordingly, about a year and a half after the community workers were initially funded, the health department was encouraged by the private physicians to hire a family nurse–practitioner to offer prenatal services at two field health offices run by the county health department. The nurse–practitioner referred high-risk women to the private physicians for prenatal care; county funds were made available to pay for such specialized care. In addition, the obstetrical staff at the local hospital voted to require physicians who agreed to care for high-risk indigent women with payment provided by the county to serve periodically as attending physicians in the health department prenatal clinics. This new service was soon saturated with women seeking care who had formerly remained outside the maternity system, thereby lessening the need for direct casefinding, except in some areas, such as trailer parks, occupied by exceedingly poor, socially isolated families.

Direct measures of the impact of these initiatives on, for example, trimester of registration in prenatal care are not available; however, the program reported that by 1984 the percentage of walk-ins at the local hospital (virtually the only hospital available for maternity care in the county) had fallen to 5 percent from the 1979 figure of 20 percent. Program staff believe that the availability of providers willing to accept some low-income women and the institution of new clinic services were probably the keys to this apparent change in prenatal care use, not the casefinding activities. As the program director noted, "Word of mouth makes complicated identification of patients unnecessary." Increasing social support through home visits from the outreach workers and other community changes probably also contributed to the apparent improvement in prenatal care use.

A crude cost-benefit analysis of the program was conducted. The analysis assumed that the program would provide prenatal care to 100 high-risk women per year in the county and that the cesarean section rate would be 20 percent. Annual savings from improved prenatal and intrapartum care were calculated to be one infant's life and $310,000 through reduced rates of low birthweight and maternal complications. With such figures in hand, along with those on the declining number of women arriving at the local hospital in labor having had little or no prenatal care (and evidence of a decline in the area's infant mortality rate), program leaders were able to convince both the county administrators and the private physicians of the success of the program and the need to continue and expand it. Support for the program has also grown because expenditures from the county indigency fund to cover the high costs of maternal and infant complications have decreased, probably due in part to the increased use of prenatal care by the area's poor, high-risk women.

At present, a nurse–practitioner funded by the state continues to provide prenatal care to poor women in the local health department, referring high-risk women to private physicians in the community. The county provides funding not only for the private care of high-risk women, but also for a full-time perinatal coordinator working in the community. Funds are no longer available for the casefinding and patient-advocacy services of the community workers, and these activities have therefore been discontinued.

Prenatal Care Assistance Program—New York State[6]

New York's Prenatal Care Assistance Program (PCAP), originally the Prenatal Care and Nutrition Program, resulted from pressures generated by a formal petition requesting that prenatal care be declared a public health service to be provided by the state. A report of the Children's Defense Fund showing that New York State led the nation in the percentage of nonwhite women receiving late or no prenatal care furthered the cause. In April 1984, the state legislature appropriated $7.5 million for outreach, education, prenatal care, and nutritional services for pregnant women who were not eligible for Medicaid, had no private health insurance, and whose family income was at or below 185 percent of the federally defined poverty level.

Applications for participation in the program were sought from public and private not-for-profit health care providers serving areas of the state believed to be at high risk because of their socioeconomic indicators and high rates of infant mortality and low birthweight. Forty-three providers were selected in January 1985; by July 1987, the number had grown to 88 projects, located in all 5 boroughs of New York City and 44 of the 57 upstate counties.

The PCAP has three major components. The Primary Prenatal Services component reimburses providers for prenatal and postpartum visits, diagnostic procedures, and physician or nurse–midwife deliveries. Required services include risk assessment, health education, nutrition services, psychosocial services, after-hours and emergency counseling and care, referral of high-risk patients, referral for pediatric care, and follow-up of missed visits and referrals. The Outreach and Education Services component includes dissemination of information on the importance of prenatal care, education to eliminate perceived barriers, recruitment, linkages with other community services, and follow-up of clients who miss appointments. These services are supported by grants to providers for staff and other costs. The third component is Prenatal Care Development. The state health department is attempting to develop services in areas without them and to expand services in areas with limited capacity. Thus, funds are available to support construction or renovation of service sites, purchase of equipment, and short-term costs of medical service personnel. The state hopes that by June 1988 these funds will ensure that 98 percent of its population will reside within 20 miles of a PCAP service site. Initiatives for 1987–1988 include a statewide media campaign, a community outreach worker program in selected areas, placement of health education staff in each regional office, a pilot home visitation program in four rural areas, an increase in the prenatal care and delivery service fee, and an in-depth evaluation of the PCAP by an outside consultant.

In the fiscal year beginning July 1986, more than 21,600 women were served by 88 projects in over 120 service sites. The state expects to serve more than half of the 49,000 women eligible for the program in 1987–1988. The average cost per client in the 1986–1987 fiscal year was $639.

A report on over 16,000 clients who entered care during 1985 and 1986, over 7,000 of whom had completed care, indicated that the PCAP was reaching racial and ethnic minorities (nonwhite women made up 51.1 percent of clients and Hispanics of all races totaled 47.1 percent), teenagers (19.3 percent of clients), and women at high risk (approximately 25 percent met demographic and medical risk criteria). The PCAP population was not initiating care early, however: less than 25 percent enrolled in the first trimester, and more than 18 percent delayed care until the third trimester. Nonetheless, the PCAP clients apparently "made up" for their late initiation of care, because they averaged just under nine visits.

The legislature has made available almost $26 million for fiscal year 1987–1988. Approximately $19 million is for the services component, more than $3 million for the outreach and education component, and more than $4 million for the development component.

Prevention of Low Birthweight Program— Onondaga County, New York[7]

Another example of a program focused heavily on basic system capacity is the Onondaga County Prevention of Low Birthweight Program, one of 14 related efforts in the state financed in large part by New York's Maternal and Child Health Block Grant. The program was developed with state encouragement and is being led jointly by the Onondaga County Health Department and the Department of Obstetrics and Gynecology of the State University of New York's Health Science Center. It began in June 1984 and was built in part on the area's successful effort to regionalize its perinatal services, with the assistance and leadership of the Robert Wood Johnson Foundation. Despite the many accomplishments of the regionalization process—in particular, striking reductions in infant mortality—it became apparent in the late 1970s and early 1980s that two residual problems required attention. First, the proportion of infants who were born at low birthweight was remaining relatively constant rather than declining. Second, a small but persistent proportion of pregnant women was receiving late (third trimester) or no prenatal care. A public health nursing survey revealed that, although late registration had some motivational and socioeconomic roots, inadequate capacity of the prenatal care system kept out even those indigent pregnant women who applied for early care.

Onondaga County statistics showed that in 1982 76 percent of pregnant women in the county obtained prenatal care in the private sector, primarily through private physicians and an HMO (health maintenance organization). According to data from the local university and health department, women who used the private sector initiated care early (94 percent in the first trimester) and faced only a 1- to 2-week lag between an appointment request and the first prenatal visit. Patients using the area's four clinics (two hospital clinics, one school-based clinic, and one neighborhood health center), however, initiated care later, due in part to a 4- to 8-week lag between an appointment request and the first visit. State vital statistics for 1981 showed that 84.6 percent of all Onondaga County residents registered in the first trimester of their pregnancy, whereas the corresponding percentage for black clients, who were more likely to use a clinic, was only 56.4 percent. An analysis of the prenatal patients registered in the clinics in August 1983 revealed that only 24 percent had been registered in their first trimester. In addition, data for 1981 from the special Supplemental Food Program for Women, Infants, and Children (WIC) showed that only 14 percent of recipients entered WIC in the first trimester, reflecting the delay of entry into medical care.

Thirty-three census tracts in the central city of Syracuse were identified as contributing disproportionately to the county's high rates of low birthweight and late registration in prenatal care. A variety of efforts was made to encourage pregnant women in this target area to begin prenatal care early in pregnancy. For example, television spots directed at the target population were developed and aired; these stressed the benefits of early prenatal care and its role in reducing low birthweight. Public awareness efforts noted the possible availability of financial support for prenatal care and encouraged women to seek care regardless of their financial status. The county health department also intensified its emphasis on the importance of prenatal care in its communication with other agencies and clients in the target area. Training sessions were held for clinic personnel serving large numbers of women from the target area; these explained ways to make clients feel more welcome and to arrange clinic procedures so that clients had shorter, more pleasant encounters.

The major emphasis, however, was on increasing the number of prenatal appointment slots, particularly for new patients. Two strategies were pursued. First, existing sites in the target area providing a large proportion of services to clinic patients (such as the Syracuse Community Health Center and the Health Science Center's Maternity Center) were provided with additional nurse–practitioner staff so that patient load could be increased. Second, three new satellite pregnancy diagnosis and triage sites were established in census tracts having especially high rates of low birthweight and low use of prenatal care. These new sites offer the full range of services usually provided at a first prenatal visit, including a history, physical examination, laboratory tests, and risk assessment. When appropriate, application for Medicaid and WIC is begun. A pregnant woman typically makes only one visit to a satellite site and is then referred elsewhere for ongoing care (primarily to the four clinics), depending on her risk status, place of residence, preferences, and similar factors. Staff spend significant amounts of time helping patients secure other needed services; in particular, patients are helped to get prompt appointments for continuing prenatal care at the facilities to which they have been referred.

The satellite clinics offer appointments within a week or two of a request (at present, because of the popularity of these satellites, waiting times for appointments are lengthening), and the appointments are free—two attributes not shared by any other public facilities in the targeted area. Each satellite clinic operates a half-day a week and is staffed by a nurse–practitioner with physician backup, a public health nurse, and a community health aide. These individuals work in the preexisting clinics during the rest of the week, thereby increasing the clinics' capacity. Anecdotal reports suggest that these teams are especially effective in developing good rapport with the clients, in scheduling adequate time for visits, and in referring clients successfully for ongoing care.

Two different data sets suggest that these improvements in the capacity of the prenatal care system have increased the proportion of pregnant women in the high-risk, target census tracts who begin prenatal care in the first trimester. The first data set spans July 1984 to July 1987 and is composed of 1,290 women residing in the target area who were subsequently identified as being at high risk for a low birthweight delivery. For this group, the average lag time between the call for a first prenatal care appointment and the appointment itself was 4.6 weeks during the first year of the program (1984), declining to 1.9 in 1987.

A second measure of impact is derived from comparisons of trimester of registration for prenatal care for all births in the target area versus all other births in the county (so-called nontarget area births). A trend analysis shows a highly statistically significant increase in the percentage of births to first-trimester registrants residing in the target area—from 71.5 percent in 1983 (before the program began in 1984) to 76.4 percent in 1986, compared to an increase of only 1 percent in the nontargeted census tracts during the same period. This general trend was apparent for white women, nonwhite women, women age 17 and under, and women age 20 and over. For 18- and 19-year-olds, the difference was larger. In 1983, 52.8 percent began prenatal care in the first trimester; in 1986, 66 percent did so, a statistically significant change. In the nontargeted area, the figure remained essentially stable at about 60 percent. The impact in the targeted census tracts was great enough to increase the county's total of first-trimester registration in prenatal care from 81.6 percent in 1983 to 85.8 percent in 1986.

Unfortunately, during these same years there was no reduction in the percentages of women receiving late or no prenatal care, suggesting that expanding the capacity of prenatal services cannot, by itself, solve the problem of nonparticipation. At present, the project is focusing its efforts on drawing this hard-to-reach population into care.

TYPE 3: PROGRAMS TO IMPROVE INSTITUTIONAL PRACTICES

In this section are summaries of six programs that try to draw more women into prenatal care by improving the nature and organization of services themselves: two Maternity and Infant Care (MIC) Projects, one in Cleveland, Ohio, and the other in three North Carolina counties; an Improved Pregnancy Outcome (IPO) Project in two counties in North

Carolina; an Improved Child Health Project (ICHP) in two areas of Mississippi; the Child Survival Project of the Presbyterian Medical Center in the city of New York; and the development of a perinatal system in Shelby County, Tennessee.

Maternity and Infant Care Projects—Ohio[8] and North Carolina[9]

The Maternity and Infant Care (MIC) Projects began in 1963 as a demonstration program administered by the federal Children's Bureau (whose health programs are now within the Bureau of Maternal and Child Health). The data produced by the projects funded in the 1960s suggested that accessible, high-quality maternity care could reduce the rate of infant mortality. In 1974 every state was required to have at least one such project, and responsibility for the projects was shifted to the states. According to a 1975 federal publication, MIC Projects not only provided medical care to pregnant women and their infants, but also provided social services, nutritional counseling, patient education, home visits by a project nurse, special services to pregnant adolescents, transportation, and child care. The projects were also to emphasize the importance of "humanizing the clinics." The description of this approach is, unfortunately, just as pertinent today as it was 12 years ago:

The most important task that each project must accomplish to reach the community is to overcome the unfavorable impression that many people have about what they can expect in the way of meaningful help from a public clinic. The women who come to the project for assistance must be sure that they will not be faced with long waits in dingy hallways on uncomfortable benches, and that they will not be rushed through treatment in assembly line fashion.[10]

Examples of humanizing include seeing the same obstetrician and public health nurse at each visit, avoiding across-the-desk interviews by using round tables, having interpreters available, and, in Atlanta, having "all new personnel . . . register as new obstetric patients on their first day of employment and 'go through the clinic.' This experience increases their awareness of what a patient's average day involves and underlines the importance of treating patients with respect and courtesy."[11]

The MIC Project at the Cleveland Metropolitan Hospital—still in operation—used many of these approaches during a period in which prenatal care utilization was studied. It operated five satellite clinics and provided social service assessments and interventions, health education, nutritional counseling, home visits, special services for adolescents, and follow-up of missed appointments.

The project tried in particular to improve the nature of the services from the clients' perspective. A patient advocacy group was formed to act as an ombudsman. A "Friends of the MIC" group was formed, with three subcommittees: Finders, who found clothes, bassinets, and other items needed by patients; Go-Getters, who provided transportation; and Rockers, who played with and rocked young children in clinics while their mothers made their prenatal visits. Training for staff was provided, to increase their sensitivity to patient needs and to possible cultural barriers between staff and clients; continuity of care was increased; and small changes in procedures were made to demonstrate a caring attitude toward patients (for example, securing parking spaces near the hospital for pregnant clinic patients). The project also mounted an intensive promotional campaign aimed at encouraging early entry into prenatal care. The campaign was staffed by 12 community workers and included door-to-door canvassing; explicit encouragement of word-of-mouth referrals (enrolled clients were asked to bring in pregnant friends and relatives); Koffee Klatches in housing projects and elsewhere, during which the MIC Project was explained; and free pregnancy testing with immediate referral of those testing positive to prenatal care.

A formal evaluation of program impact on various measures of outcome was conducted by comparing more than 3,000 mothers who received MIC care in 1976 and 1977 with approximately half that number who received care and delivered at the same hospital but who were ineligible for MIC care because they resided outside the target area. The MIC and comparison groups were similar on numerous sociodemographic measures, but the MIC group had higher levels of medical and obstetric risk. The rates of early registration for care were significantly higher in the MIC group (MIC: first trimester, 47.6 percent; first half of pregnancy, 69.0 percent; non-MIC: first trimester, 34.0 percent; first half of pregnancy, 56.5 percent).

Project staff report that many of these service improvements were not sustained beyond the 1970s. The 12 community workers, for example, were decreased to 4 by 1979. In recent years, rates of early registration in prenatal care have reportedly decreased.

The MIC Project in North Carolina operated in three rural counties. Its services included active casefinding, transportation, public health nursing, nutrition and social services, health education, and follow-up of missed appointments. Participants between 1970 and 1977 were compared to similar residents in three other counties during the same period. The two sets of women were quite comparable, but there were some significant differences, including higher risk for inadequate prenatal care in the MIC group. Compared to the control group, the MIC population was more heavily nonwhite, unmarried, and less educated. Nonetheless, the MIC group exhibited a smaller proportion of women with inadequate care (Kessner index definition) than did the comparison group. Moreover, when five risk factors were held constant in the analysis (the three already mentioned plus two measures of obstetric risk), a larger proportion of the MIC group than of the comparison group received quantitatively adequate care (Kessner index definition).

Improved Pregnancy Outcome Project—Two Counties in North Carolina[12]

The federal Improved Pregnancy Outcome (IPO) Project began in 1976. States with high rates of infant mortality received funds to "improve maternal care and pregnancy outcomes." States were given considerable freedom to design their IPO programs, though improving organizational arrangements was emphasized at the federal level. For its IPO Project, North Carolina chose a two-county project site that was disproportionately rural and poor, with excessive rates of perinatal and infant mortality. Prenatal and maternity resources in the area were extremely limited. Funds were used to increase maternity services by having certified nurse–midwives provide maternity care, with obstetric backup, and to expand health department services to include social services, health education, and nutrition counseling. The program also featured casefinding and transportation, directed particularly at teenagers and others at high risk.

The project was evaluated by comparing the experience of IPO registrants to that of all women in the IPO counties (including the registrants) and to women in several neighboring counties judged to be roughly comparable in health care resources and in both socioeconomic and perinatal status. Evaluation was confined to black women. In 1972–1976, before the project began, about 27 percent of black women in the IPO counties and 19.5 percent of black women in the comparison counties received quantitatively adequate prenatal care (defined by a modified version of the Kessner index). By 1979–1981, during which time the project was operating and the evaluation data collected, 49.6 of black women in the IPO counties and 41.2 percent of IPO registrants received adequate care versus 30.3 percent of black women in the comparison counties.

Improved Child Health Project—Two Areas of Mississippi[13]

The federal Improved Child Health Projects (ICHP) were initiated in 1978 to improve pregnancy outcomes and followed the same pattern as the IPO Projects, although a portion of the funds was to be used for in-hospital care. In Mississippi, two projects were funded (ICHP #1 and ICHP #2), each of which covered several counties. In general, the funds were used to add staff to health departments and to provide transportation, social services, tracking, and casefinding services. High-risk referral centers were also established.

The project was evaluated using several comparison groups. The results were mixed. In one set of ICHP counties, the percentage of all women with quantitatively adequate care (using a modified Kessner index definition) increased 14.6 percent between 1975–1978 and 1979–1981, while in the comparison counties it increased by only 9.2 percent. In a second set of ICHP counties, the percentage of all women with adequate care increased 3.5 percent over the same interval but increased even more—8.7 percent— in the control counties. The evaluators believe this is because the first group of counties used a community-planning approach involving both public and private providers, while the second group of counties had problems in implementa- tion, resulting in, among other things, less success in reaching target populations.

Child Survival Project, Columbia–Presbyterian Medical Center—New York City[14]

Columbia–Presbyterian Medical Center (CPMC) serves the Washington Heights neighborhood of New York City, an area with a large Hispanic population and high rates of poverty and teenage pregnancy. Many residents in 1982 were newly arrived immigrants, including an unknown number who were in the United States illegally. Lack of knowledge about the health care system, lack of English-language skills, and significant financial constraints posed serious obstacles to the use of health services generally, and timely prenatal care in particular. Data from the New York City Department of Health revealed that in 1982 28 percent of women in the community received late or no prenatal care.

A grant from the Child Survival/Fair Start Program of the Ford Foundation to the Center for Population and Family Health of the Columbia University School of Public Health financed a program from 1982 to 1985 to reduce the percentage of community women receiving inadequate prenatal care. Other program goals included improving infant feeding practices (specifically, encouraging breast-feeding) and bolstering the use of health care services during the first years of life. The program pursued a complex blend of activities within the Medical Center and within the community as well, trying in particular to strengthen links between the two. Within the community, for example, the program used volunteers and existing networks to call attention to issues of maternal and child health and to disseminate information to pregnant women and new mothers on such topics as the elements of well-baby care and where to go for checkups. In general, the program leaders found that the institutional changes they accomplished within the hospital were more easily measured and probably more successful than the more diffuse efforts in the community. Two of the hospital-based activities are summarized here: an effort to shorten the time between confirmation of pregnancy and first prenatal visit, and making the Medicaid certification process less complex.

To speed entry into prenatal care, the Child Survival Team arranged for a nurse–midwife and a bilingual health advocate to be placed in the hospital's pregnancy screening clinic. The nurse–midwife counseled all women about the need for prenatal care and healthful behavior during pregnancy and also screened and referred women at high risk for poor pregnancy outcomes. In addition, the obstetrics department agreed to designate all women age 18 and under or who first visited the clinic in their third trimester as high risk and thus immediately eligible for prenatal care, regardless of ability to pay. The health advocate guided patients through the process of making an appointment for prenatal services, which was especially difficult for women who spoke little or no English. In addition, the appointment system for financial screening, laboratory services, and the initial visit was centralized, and the number of appointments for financial screening and prenatal care was increased.

With regard to Medicaid, it was clear that the certification process was a major block to care, since an appointment for an initial prenatal visit could not be made until the pregnant woman actually had a Medicaid card. The process was made particularly difficult because the city's Medicaid application form had not been translated into Spanish. In addition, the Medicaid Eligibility Unit at the hospital had been limited to inpatient care. Agreement was reached to hire a bilingual staff member to work in the outpatient obstetric clinic. This worker saw women the same day they had a positive pregnancy test, assisted them in completing the Medicaid application form and in obtaining the necessary documentation, made appointments at the city Medicaid office, and helped resolve problems that arose in the application process. Efforts to get the application form translated into Spanish were successful. Additional changes included the employment of a liaison person to hand carry the completed Medicaid applications to the Medicaid office, correct mistakes, and obtain a Medicaid number. The hospital also agreed to allow prenatal appointments to be made for women who had been notified in writing that their Medicaid application had been accepted but who had not yet received their Medicaid card. And finally, a reduced-rate prenatal package, payable in installments, was introduced for women ineligible for Medicaid.

These several institutional reforms reduced the delay in obtaining a first prenatal appointment from up to 90 days after the positive pregnancy test to about 2 weeks. According to the program's leaders, the improvements in bureaucratic process, coupled with such other program elements as the placement of a bilingual health advocate in the prenatal clinics and the community-level health education initiatives alluded to earlier, led to increased patient understanding of and satisfaction with prenatal care. Most of the system improvements have remained in place.

The team leader traces the project's success to the involvement of the bureaucracy in the process of change and the ability of the Child Survival team to show that not only did community women benefit from the program, but so did the medical center. The overall costs of the changes to the hospital, especially additional staff, were substantially reduced by the increased volume of visits and more timely Medicaid reimbursements, since more women were found eligible for Medicaid and began making visits earlier. However, detailed cost computations are not available.

Development of a Perinatal System in Shelby County, Tennessee[15]

In 1977 the Department of Obstetrics and Gynecology at the University of Tennessee established a Division of Ambulatory and Community Medicine and recruited two faculty members whose charge was to convert fragmented services in Memphis and Shelby County into a smoothly functioning system of perinatal services for women relying on care provided in publicly financed settings. At the time, prenatal care for these women was fragmented among health department clinics, hospital clinics, and grant-funded neighborhood health centers, and there were 6- to 8-week delays for a first prenatal appointment at the county hospital clinic. Although all deliveries occurred at the county hospital, there was little communication of patient information among the various facilities, no standardized prenatal record, and deteriorating attitudes toward patients among personnel at the clinic. As a result of these problems and others, the infant mortality rate within the area was over 20 deaths per 1,000 live births, and many patients who had not received care or for whom no record of care was available came to the county hospital for delivery.

The providers, including the medical faculty and the staffs of the county hospital and the health department, developed a plan to integrate the facilities into a coordinated perinatal care system. The initial risk assessment at the county hospital clinic was continued, but all low-risk patients were referred to the health department clinics for ongoing care; a standard prenatal record was adopted; an improved appointment system was instituted; and obstetrical faculty were assigned to all prenatal clinics in the county hospital, with the goal of changing the attitudes and behavior of the providers in those settings. In order to improve the quality of care, the number of health department clinics was reduced from 12 to 6, allowing each clinic to be staffed by specially trained nurses, and a 1-month training program and protocol were developed for the health department nurses who provided prenatal care. These programs were subsequently expanded to include three adjoining rural counties under the asupices of the Robert Wood Johnson Foundation's Rural Infant Care Program.

From 1980 to 1985, the percentage of women delivering at the county hospital who initiated care in the first trimester increased from 16 to 23 percent, and the percentage with no prenatal care decreased from 26 to 14 percent. According to the project director, other results included a reduction in the time between initial call and first appointment from 6 weeks to 5 days at the county hospital clinic, an increase in the percentage of patients enrolled in the system whose records were available at time of delivery (from 40 to 95 percent), improved skills among the nurses in health department clinics, and improved attitudes among providers in the county hospital clinic.

TYPE 4: PROGRAMS THAT CONDUCT CASEFINDING

Ten examples of casefinding for prenatal care were studied by the Committee. The Central Harlem Outreach Program and the Community Health Advocacy Program of New York City have collected data on the casefinding effectiveness of outreach workers. The Better Babies Project of Washington, D.C., and the Maternity and Infant Outreach Project of Hartford, Connecticut, employ a wide variety of casefinding techniques, including outreach workers. Three hotlines were studied—the Pregnancy Healthline in New York City, 961-BABY in Detroit, and CHOICE in Philadelphia. Two examples of casefinding through referrals among programs were assessed—a Tulsa, Oklahoma, project that provided free pregnancy testing coupled with volunteer advocates linking pregnant women to prenatal care, and a set of studies that examine the role of WIC nutrition programs in recruiting pregnant women into prenatal care. Finally, the Committee reviewed a recent baby shower project in Michigan, a type of incentive-oriented effort to recruit women into prenatal care.

Central Harlem Outreach Program—New York City[16]

The Central Harlem Outreach Program operated between August 1, 1982, and September 30, 1983. It was financed by the Commonwealth Fund to develop and test strategies that might decrease perinatal and early childhood morbidity in a group of urban, low-income mothers and infants. Central Harlem is home to a group of economically deprived black families whose rates of inadequate prenatal care, adolescent pregnancy, low birthweight, and infant mortality are significantly higher than those of the city as a whole.

The program had three components: an outreach program designed to identify pregnant women early in their pregnancies and enroll them in care in the Harlem Hospital system; a travel allowance for enrolled women during pregnancy and their infant's first year to encourage compliance with prenatal and child care; and a group of community workers—"maternal advocates"—to provide basic health information and social support during pregnancy and the first year postpartum. Only the first component will be described.

Four outreach workers (ORWs) were employed to locate pregnant women not in prenatal care and recruit them into the Harlem Hospital system. All were community residents, had extensive social networks, were unemployed, and seemed comfortable on the street. They were supervised by a social worker who was also a community resident. The ORWs met twice a week with the supervisor to discuss strategies for finding pregnant women. The ORWs were paid a small commission ($10) for each pregnant woman they found who entered the Harlem Hospital system. In addition, the ORWs received a salary, but it was less than that of comparable workers in the hospital.

The ORWs reported using a variety of strategies. They began by advertising the program. They designed flyers and placed them where women would see them. They spent most of their time in welfare offices and clinic settings, but they also did door-to-door canvassing in apartment buildings and approached women on the streets. Casefinding in apartment buildings and housing projects yielded few contacts, because fear of crime has led to mistrust of door-to-door canvassers.

The outreach program was carefully evaluated. In 1 year, three full-time-equivalent ORWs (there was some attrition) made approximately 7,400 contacts, an estimated 20 contacts per day. They located 285 pregnant women, of whom 104 were not receiving prenatal care. Only half of these enrolled in a Harlem Hospital facility. Women who enrolled as a result of outreach contact started care slightly earlier than those who did not (at 15.8 versus 17.0 weeks). They were more likely to be 20 or older, to live with a husband or boyfriend, and to have experienced a prior adverse outcome of pregnancy.

The outreach component of the program cost approximately $44,000, including all of the ORWs and one-third of the supervisor's salaries, incentive payments to the ORWs, and miscellaneous expenses. Thus, the cost was $6 per contact; $155 per pregnant woman located; $440 per potential enrollee; and $846 per actual enrollee. The program staff were not convinced that this was a cost-effective way to encourage enrollment in the Harlem Hospital system of prenatal care.

Community Health Advocacy Program—New York City[17]

Before its efforts within the Presbyterian Medical Center (see the description of the Child Survival Project, above), the Center for Population and Family Health implemented a community-based project to link high-risk women and adolescents to prenatal and other reproductive health services. This Community Health Advocacy Program was supported by federal and state agencies and a consortium of private foundations and was designed to train bilingual (Spanish and English) community residents, called health advocates, to provide preventive health education, referral, and counseling services in homes and other community sites. Social area analysis was used to identify those census tracts in the Washington Heights community that had had high rates of poor birth outcomes over the preceding several years. The program focused on finding individuals in the target area who do not often use preventive services without special encouragement or assistance and linking them to services at the Columbia–Presbyterian Medical Center and other health care sites in the city. The program stressed contraception, prenatal care, and general concepts of reproductive health. Volunteers were used to supplement the casefinding and health education work of the salaried health advocates.

Over an 18-month period (April 1981 to September 1982), 979 men and women became registered clients of the program; that is, they allowed an advocate to discuss health and social services needs with them, received referrals, general counseling, and advocacy support as appropriate, and agreed to be contacted again for follow-up. Of the 979 clients, 72 women (7 percent) were either pregnant or possibly pregnant. Of the 72, 32 were already receiving pregnancy-related services; thus, only 40 of all individuals contacted (4 percent) were in need of prenatal care. All of these women were referred to prenatal services by the health advocate, but 13 did not go to the site to which they were referred. Larger numbers of women, especially teenagers and older women, were located who needed other reproductive health services, but follow-up data suggest that more than half the referrals for such services were unsuccessful. Follow-up information on over 60 percent of the referrals, however, was not available.

The program leader has suggested several reasons that might account for the limited impact. First, the project's evaluation design prevented the program from expanding beyond an initial 10-block area, even though it soon became clear that the number of persons in need of services who could be contacted by an advocate was very low. Second, although most of the community residents were from the Dominican Republic, many of the health advocates and volunteers that assisted in the door-to-door canvassing were from other ethnic groups, raising issues of cultural incompatibility. In particular, a large proportion of community residents were newly arrived immigrants (an unknown proportion of whom were in the United States illegally) who might have been suspicious of representatives from a formal institution.

A high rate of staff and volunteer turnover limited the ability of the program to sustain a consistent image in the target areas, and over time many volunteers left for paying jobs, particularly those who were more highly skilled. (Some approaches to recruiting, training, and maintaining volunteers, however, were found to be useful and have been described thoughtfully in a final program summary submitted to funders.) This underlying instability was compounded by the fact that the target communities were themselves highly mobile; 54 percent of program clients had been in the community less than 5 years, and moves within the neighborhood were frequent. Security problems increased program costs, since staff would work only in pairs and canvassing had to be limited to daylight hours.

It also became apparent that other concerns, such as jobs, housing, and instruction in English, were of much greater importance to neighborhood residents than preventive health care. In response to this finding, the project made several modifications in its approach. For example, the staff developed a series of pamphlets on health maintenance that were used in English-as-a-second-language classes in the community as a part of the Child Survival Project described earlier.

The Better Babies Project—Washington, D.C.[18]

The Better Babies Project (BBP) is an intervention program that is attempting to reduce the incidence of low birthweight by 20 percent in nine contiguous census tracts in the District of Columbia; the population in this area is largely black and poor. Begun in 1986, the project is to be completed in 1990, after which point its impact on low birthweight will be assessed. Several comparison groups have been defined, and a sophisticated evaluation is planned with the assistance of the National Institute of Child Health and Human Development.

BBP employs many methods to locate pregnant women in the target area and enroll them in the program. Once in the program, women are linked to prenatal services, if they are not already in care (most are); their risks for low birthweight are assessed; and an individual treatment plan is developed and carried out to address those risks. Most enrollees—known as participants—are in monthly, often weekly, contact with the program.

BBP includes a casefinding staff of 10 and a drop-in center. Eight Service Coordinators, under the supervision of two Service Supervisors, are responsible for casefinding, using neighborhood canvassing and other techniques, and for providing health education and friendly support at the drop-in center and in participants' homes. Multiple types of canvassing are used. Service Coordinators are assigned areas and given logs, maps, and lists of addresses to improve their efficiency. In each area, they stop women, men, and children on the street to tell them about BBP, asking women to come to the drop-in center if they are pregnant and asking everyone to pass the message to friends who are pregnant. Carrying bright yellow canvas bags with large BBP emblems, they systematically knock on household doors and talk to anyone who responds, selectively leaving buttons, key chains, or refrigerator magnets as reminders. A BBP pamphlet or flyer is slid under the door when there is no answer and is handed selectively to people met at home or on the street. As safety measures, the Service Coordinators usually work in pairs, occasionally attend the police roll call, and carry boat sirens to use in an emergency.

Service Coordinators also visit local businesses and bring the message of the importance of prenatal care to owners and salespeople, always including a request to refer pregnant women to BBP. By special arrangement, recruiting also takes place in the waiting rooms of several public and private clinics. BBP has attempted telephone canvassing, but did not find it very productive. Some poor households do not have phones. When the caller does reach a low-income household, the number of women recruited is low, since pregnancy is not that common, even when pregnancy among friends is included. BBP staff note, however, that telephone canvassing is often the only way to reach women who do not leave their homes and will not answer the door. The phone is also used regularly to canvass former participants and staff members' personal networks in the community. Service Coordinators spend approximately 20 percent of their time in casefinding and the remainder in offering specific interventions (such as help in smoking reduction) in participants' homes or the drop-in center and in providing friendly support.

Third-party referrals are also sought by staff. Service Supervisors maintain contact with WIC and welfare offices, EPSDT (the Early and Periodic Screening, Diagnosis and Treatment Program of Medicaid) staff, school personnel, clergy, social service agencies, day care centers, women's groups, soup kitchens, battered women's shelters, and private physicians. The program has two public service radio announcements that are aired occasionally. Staff also participate periodically in local radio talk shows.

The drop-in center, which functions primarily as a base for social support and intervention activities, also assists in casefinding. Its visibility reminds pregnant women of the need for care and provides a place where they can receive help in selecting a source of prenatal care and obtaining an appointment. The center offers free pregnancy testing; women who have positive tests are guided immediately to a prenatal care provider, as appropriate. Women using the center for group activities, snacks and light meals, or rest often inform the staff of pregnancies among relatives and friends.

BBP uses cash and other participation incentives. A $10 monthly stipend is offered to women who keep their prenatal appointments. A woman can receive a maximum of between $50 and $100, depending on how early in her pregnancy she enrolls. The money is intended to help defray costs associated with prenatal care, such as transportation to appointments, medications, and child care. Moreover, anyone who successfully refers a pregnant woman to BBP receives $5 for the referral. The BBP staff believes that the financial incentive is not viewed by participants as being as important as the friendly support from the Service Coordinators and the availability of the drop-in center in enrolling women and sustaining their participation.

Data will not be available until late 1991 on the impact of the program on low birthweight. Preliminary data are available, however, on the characteristics of women enrolled in the program between January 1, 1986, and March 31, 1987, and on the yield of specific casefinding efforts. Of 520 women contacted and believed to be eligible for enrollment (that is, believed to be less than 32 weeks pregnant and a resident of the target area), 66 percent were already in prenatal care, 30 percent were not, and 4 percent were not certain they were pregnant. Of the women enrolled in the program, 64 percent were between 0 and 20 weeks pregnant; 78 percent entered prenatal care between 0 and 21 weeks. Those not in care at the time of initial contact were earlier in their pregnancies than those already in care.

Referrals came from a wide variety of sources: 30 percent from neighborhood and door-to-door canvassing, 22 percent from friends and relatives, 15 percent from clinics and hospitals, and 12 percent from other participants; 10 percent were walk-ins with no specific referral source. Telephone surveys and the media advertisements yielded about 3 percent of referrals. The rest were from a variety of sources, including one referral from the District's Commissioner of Public Health.

Information is also available on the source of referral for participants who are pregnant and already in prenatal care versus those who are pregnant but not yet in care. As expected, clinics and hospitals generate more program participants who are in care than not, but otherwise the relative yield of various referral sources is about the same for both groups. In 1986, 44 percent of enrolled women already in care were referred by a friend, relative, or other participant or were walk-ins with no referral source; 17 percent were referred by a clinic or hospital; 31 percent came from neighborhood canvassing; and the rest came from other sources. For pregnant women not in care, referral sources were 47 percent from a friend, relative, or other participant or were walk-ins; 5 percent were from a clinic or hospital; 36 percent from neighborhood canvassing; and the rest were from other sources.

The Maternity and Infant Outreach Project—Hartford, Connecticut[19]

The Hartford Action Plan on Infant Health was developed in the early 1980s in response to the city's very high rate of infant mortality. It was spearheaded by a consortium of corporate leaders, including representatives of banks and insurance companies. The Maternity and Infant Outreach Project (MIOP) is one of the Action Plan's components and was built on the experience of the city's Improved Pregnancy Outcome Project and longstanding Maternity and Infant Care Project. Like the Better Babies Project in Washington, MIOP does not provide prenatal care directly, but rather offers services that supplement medical care. These services include social support, counseling on nutrition, help in securing welfare and housing assistance, and assistance with substance abuse problems, often through home visiting. Program participants are followed through the first 6 months of the baby's life. Seven neighborhoods with high rates of infant mortality were targeted when MIOP began in July 1985. As of December 31, 1987, 1,057 women have been enrolled in the program, which is housed in the Hartford City Health Department and is funded by both private and public donors. The seven neighborhoods were divided into three areas, and a team composed of a health educator and two neighborhood health workers was assigned to each area. The workers try to recruit pregnant women into care and to provide social support.

MIOP has collected data on referral sources and on the yield of its casefinding activities. About 40 percent of MIOP clients are referred to the program by community clinics and by the obstetric clinics in the three Hartford hospitals. These women are already in prenatal care but are referred to MIOP because the clinic providers judge them to be at high risk of a poor pregnancy outcome or difficulties postpartum, or both. Defined risk factors include social isolation, being 16 or younger, a history of social or emotional problems, and a previous preterm delivery. Seventeen percent are referred by family planning clinics, and 36 percent are referred through such MIOP casefinding activities as street and door-to-door canvassing, group discussions in community settings, media announcements, and the efforts of neighborhood Baby Watch volunteers. Street and door-to-door canvassing was the most successful of these casefinding methods, yielding 16 percent of program participants. Self-referral or other clients accounted for 12 percent of referral sources. Media spots, Baby Watch volunteers, and referrals from other neighborhood organizations each yielded very few participants.

MIOP has specifically examined the methods most successful in locating pregnant women not already in prenatal care and has concluded that family planning clinics are key referral sources. Forty-three percent of MIOP participants who were in their first trimester of pregnancy but not in care were first identified through the health department's family planning clinic. Street canvassing and door-to-door inquiries yielded 25 percent of this group; self-referral accounted for 10 percent. More than half (54 percent) of MIOP clients not in care who were in the second trimester of pregnancy were referred by the family planning clinic, and 23 percent were identified via street canvassing and door-to-door work. For women in the third trimester, the family planning clinic remained the most successful referral source. In light of these data, increased efforts are being made to recruit clients through family planning systems. The project director reports that threats of violence and general security concerns are forcing them to decrease street and door-to-door canvassing, even though these methods, too, seem effective.

The program costs approximately $430,000 per year. The community workers receive about $17,000 annually. No evaluation of the project has been completed that relates costs to the number of clients found by the casefinding work.

MIOP does not know whether its casefinding and advocacy are leading to earlier registration and continuation in prenatal care. Although first-trimester registration rates increased in five of the seven targeted neighborhoods between 1985 and 1986 (from 48.8 percent to 52.3 percent; MIOP began in July 1985), comparison data from other neighborhoods have not been analyzed, and specially constituted comparison groups have not been defined.

Pregnancy Healthline—New York City[20]

The Pregnancy Healthline (PHL) is an ongoing project of the New York City Health Department, part of a mayoral initiative to decrease both infant mortality and the percentage of women who receive late or no prenatal care. The Healthline number is answered by a PHL staff member from 9:00 a.m. to 5:00 p.m., Monday through Friday. After 5:00 p.m. and on weekends and city holidays, a recorded message instructs callers to leave a number at which their call can be returned. All PHL staff are female. Their education varies from a high school degree through master's training. Several are bilingual, and two are trilingual. All are trained in women's health issues.

The PHL goes beyond the usual question-answering and referral functions of a hotline. In particular, it is able to schedule prenatal appointments during the initial call to the hotline. Over 70 facilities give PHL blocks of appointments into which hotline staff can schedule callers, saving them a second phone call. PHL only negotiates appointment blocks with facilities that can provide appointments within 2 weeks. Before making an appointment, PHL staff obtains financial information. If a woman is eligible for Medicaid, she is sent to a facility that can do Medicaid eligibility on site. Staff members also conduct a rudimentary risk assessment in order to refer women to the most appropriate facility or to obtain additional help for them.

Staff members contact the prenatal care facilities weekly to give them appointment information and to determine which PHL-referred women did not keep appointments the previous week (33 percent in 1986). The PHL staff attempts to contact these women (successfully in about 40 percent of the cases) to determine why the appointments were not kept and to assist women in overcoming obstacles to obtaining care. Many have sought care on their own at other sites; some had miscarriages or abortions. For a few, PHL staff make another prenatal appointment. In addition, the staff attempts to contact 30 percent of women who keep their appointments, stratified by risk status, to determine whether they have continued in care, to assess satisfaction with care, and, if they have delivered, to learn the outcome of the pregnancy. This process also uncovers problems which the staff tries to overcome by becoming client advocates in the health care system.

The Healthline uses a variety of techniques to make its services known. It was launched with a mass media campaign that included television and radio spots, subway cards, posters, flyers, and wallet cards. The program has also advertised in local and citywide newspapers, as well as in telephone directories for particular boroughs and for New York's Spanish-speaking population. PHL staff have established relationships with other agencies that work with similar populations, presented them with information on the Healthline, and cooperated with them on direct mailings that display the phone number prominently. PHL announcements have been included in welfare check and Medicaid mailings. It is also advertised through the Women's Health Program (another part of the mayoral infant mortality reduction initiative), which employs health educators who offer educational sessions in the target areas and promote the Healthline. In addition, the project sends a newsletter to women who keep their appointments. PHL tests its media ideas using focus groups, and it has found that subway ads in particular increase the number of calls. Radio spots and telephone directory listings have been found useful, more so than television spots. The PHL phone number has also appeared in media campaigns developed by other groups, including the New York chapter of the March of Dimes, the Mayor's Office of Adolescent Pregnancy and Parenting Services, and the New York State Family Planning Media Consortium.

From its inception in February 1985 through the end of September 1987, PHL received over 51,000 calls. In the last 9-month period for which data have been analyzed (January through September 1987), more than 20,000 calls were received. More than half of the calls (63 percent) were pregnancy-related, and another large group concerned family planning, abortion, and various gynecological problems. Sociodemographic data on the callers suggest that they are at high risk for low use of prenatal care. Sixteen percent of the callers were under 18 years old; 9 percent had health insurance, about 16 percent were on Medicaid, and 76 percent had no health insurance at all.

Between February 1985 and January 1986, over half the callers, especially women without the proper immigration papers and the working poor, cited financial problems as barriers to care, and over 10 percent had difficulty securing care due to a recent move. Some of these were homeless women who had been placed in welfare hotels in unfamiliar neighborhoods. The staff rated 18.4 percent of the women as being at medical risk, 21 percent at social risk, and 4 percent as both.

The 961-BABY Telephone Information and Referral Service—Detroit, Michigan[21]

961-BABY is a 24-hour telephone information and referral service. It was established in 1984 by the Detroit–Wayne County Infant Health Promotion Coalition, which is composed of 42 agencies. Telephones are answered by professional counselors who are trained to manage crisis situations as well as to provide information about health and social services. Callers are given the names, locations, and telephone numbers of appropriate agencies; appointments are not made. 961-BABY refers women only to prenatal facilities that can provide psychosocial and nutritional services, health education, postpartum care, family planning, and well-baby care. The facility must be able to offer care within 10 business days of an appointment request and not ask initially about source of payment for care. Callers are asked if they will allow the staff to call them back to determine whether they followed through on the referral and whether they were satisfied with the care that they received.

Like New York's Pregnancy Healthline, 961-BABY staff act as advocates for callers in securing appointments, applying for public assistance and Medicaid, and other needs. The hotline director routinely discusses with the leaders of major prenatal care providers in the area ways to improve services and to resolve the problems that hotline callers report. Project staff believe such advocacy is a critical element of a service directed at individuals likely to remain outside existing networks of health and social services.

Initially, 961-BABY depended upon public service announcements and other free publicity to advertise its presence. Commercial advertising, including television and radio spot announcements and billboards, was used for half of 1986, with positive results. Television was the most important source of information about the service for the callers, followed by radio and friends and relatives.

Since its inception, 961-BABY has received over 23,000 calls, 7,500 in 1987 alone. Each year the volume of calls grows. Forty-six percent of the calls in 1987 were related to prenatal care. Sociodemographic data suggest that the hotline is being used by women at risk of insufficient prenatal care. Almost a fifth of the callers who sought information about prenatal care in 1987 were under 18 years old, over three-quarters were black, and four-fifths were unmarried. Half called while they were still in their first trimester. The number of women calling who were Detroit residents represented about 13 percent of births in Detroit.

Recently, an attempt was made to contact a random sample of callers 4 to 6 weeks after their call to the hotline to determine whether they followed through on advice and information offered by answering staff. Only 36 percent could be located, suggesting that a substantial portion of the callers are highly mobile, which is also indicated by the demographic characteristics of callers. Of the women located, about three-fourths agreed to be interviewed by telephone. Of these, 80 percent reported that they had called to make a prenatal appointment within 1 week of the 961-BABY referral. Fifty-three percent kept that appointment; the 47 percent who did not gave a variety of reasons for not doing so. The most common were that the clinic to which they were referred was not convenient in hours or location and that the person answering the phone was rude or unfriendly. Most of these women, however, eventually secured prenatal care elsewhere. Ninety-two percent were satisfied with the help they received from the hotline counselors.

Concern for Health Options: Information, Care and Education (CHOICE)—Philadelphia, Pennsylvania[22]

CHOICE is a private, nonprofit organization in Philadelphia that conducts a variety of educational and advocacy activities on aspects of women's reproductive health. One of its functions is the operation of the CHOICE hotline, which provides counseling and referrals for family planning, prenatal care, pregnancy options, and other women's health issues. Like both of the hotlines described earlier, CHOICE uses information gained from callers to identify problems in the maternity care system and to act on behalf of individual women and for system improvements generally. A recent focus, for example, was the elimination of preadmission deposits for labor and delivery services at area hospitals.

Many activities are used to advertise the hotline, to convey various messages about reproductive health, and to inform women of Philadelphia's Maternal and Infant Care (MIC) Projects. These activities include newspaper ads and articles, subway and bus cards, listings in the white and yellow pages, public service announcements on radio and television, the distribution of consumer brochures in English and Spanish, brochures and posters for teenagers, and wallet cards. CHOICE staff appear at health fairs and on talk shows, arrange celebrity participation in various events promoting the program, make presentations at area workshops and training sessions, and support a teen theatre group. Information about the service is also sent regularly to school nurses and counselors, family planning counselors at pregnancy testing sites, and to other providers. Special informational efforts have been targeted at the Hispanic population.

From July 1, 1986, through June 30, 1987, the hotline received more than 24,000 calls. Half of these were for pregnancy testing and counseling referrals and about a quarter concerned family planning, sexually transmitted diseases, and other reproductive health issues. Among the remaining quarter were some 1,827 calls from women who knew they were pregnant, lived in Philadelphia, and wanted help in finding a prenatal care provider.

Descriptive information on these maternity care callers suggests that the hotline reached the intended audience of low-income and teenage women. Almost 40 percent of the calls were from teenagers. Of those who knew their insurance status, more than two-thirds had none and more than a fifth had Medicaid. Forty-one percent of the women who knew their pregnancy status were in the first trimester. However, only 2 percent of the calls were from Hispanic women, despite the special efforts to advertise the hotline to the Hispanic community. Over time, the hotline appears to be attracting more uninsured and teenage callers. They are also further along in pregnancy than callers several years ago, which may have some relationship to new constraints on the public financing of abortions in the state. A recent evaluation revealed that about two-thirds of the women referred to MIC projects for prenatal care actually enrolled at the sites to which they were referred.

Word-of-mouth was the most frequently cited source of information about the hotline, followed by the various public information activities noted above. The third most common source of referral to the hotline was hospitals, clinics, and agencies. Callers who knew about CHOICE through the various public information activities were reached earlier in their pregnancies than those who cited other referral sources. The staff has concluded that public information activities about the hotline were the single most effective method of reaching teenagers, uninsured women, and women in their first trimester of pregnancy—all of whom were target groups. Staff has also concluded that reaching women at high risk of insufficient prenatal care requires a clear, simple, and direct message in promotional materials.

The Free Pregnancy Testing and Prenatal Care Advocate Program—Tulsa, Oklahoma[23]

Low rates of prenatal care use and high rates of low birthweight prompted a major community effort in Tulsa County, Oklahoma, to improve pregnancy outcomes. A key element was promoting entry into prenatal care in the first trimester by providing free pregnancy tests, supplemented by volunteer patient advocates to facilitate entry into prenatal care. The project was sponsored by the Community Service Council of greater Tulsa.

The free pregnancy testing service was offered once a week at four area clinics over a 14-week period in 1987 and was advertised on local radio stations in order to reach community groups known to be at high risk of late registration in prenatal care—low-income women, black women, and teenagers, particularly black teenagers. The advertisements referred listeners to HELPLINE, a 24-hour telephone information and referral service, for specifics of where and when the free tests were available. In addition, the tests were also advertised through the newspaper and through flyers distributed in areas where women in the target groups might see them, such as housing projects. The clinics providing the tests were also asked to let callers know of the free service.

Volunteer patient advocates did the actual pregnancy testing and counseling and consulted with all women about the importance of prenatal care and about reproductive health generally. A woman testing positive who chose to seek prenatal care at one of five designated sites providing obstetric services was asked by an advocate to participate in a special project by allowing the advocate to help her arrange for prenatal care and obtain other services she might need (such as Medicaid).

During the 14 weeks of the project, 1,252 women obtained free tests at the four pregnancy testing sites. Seventy-eight percent of these women were asked how they found out about the service. Forty-three percent mentioned the radio advertisements, 25 percent the clinics themselves, 13 percent friends, and the rest a host of other sources. As a result of the radio advertisements, calls to HELPLINE for pregnancy testing and many other reproductive health services increased significantly. For example, during the project interval, 85 calls per month were made to HELPLINE for birth control and pregnancy testing services versus 7 per month over the same period a year earlier.

Data from the most popular of the four testing sites (one that performed 62 percent of the 1,252 tests) suggest that the free pregnancy testing brought more women in for testing than before the service was available. From April through July 1986, the year before the project, this site administered 795 pregnancy tests. Over those same 4 months in 1987, which include the 14-week program, 1,239 tests were completed, 774 of which were free and done as part of the special program. This represents a 56 percent increase in testing volume over the previous year. Similar data from the other three sites are not available, but program leaders report increases in these settings. Representation of black women and young women in the test population was greater than their representation in the Tulsa County childbearing population, suggesting that the targeting of the project may have been successful. However, because a demographic profile of women obtaining pregnancy tests at the four sites before the project is not available, it is not possible to determine whether the special program drew in greater numbers of women from the target groups.

A preliminary evaluation of the program has tried to assess whether the free pregnancy testing coupled with clinic-based patient advocates led to earlier registration in prenatal care, particularly among women in the target groups. Of the 1,252 tests administered over the 14 weeks of the project, results were recorded for 1,107; of these, 406 were positive. Of these 406 women, 236 (58 percent) chose not to enroll in the patient advocate program, usually due to a desire to obtain prenatal care from a private doctor or at a site other than the five participating in the special study. Of the 170 women actually enrolling in the patient advocate program, 53 withdrew from the project because of moving, miscarriage, switching to a care provider not in the project, or other reasons; 117 women continued in the project. A demographic comparison of the women who withdrew from the project and those who remained showed that the groups were quite similar in age distribution but that those who remained in the project were more likely to be white.

About 50 percent of the women who continued in the project obtained prenatal care in the first 12 weeks of pregnancy. Fifty-two percent of white women and 49 percent of black women obtained early care; among women under the age of 20, 49 percent obtained care in the first trimester.

Although no control group was constituted for a formal evaluation, program leaders did compare the prenatal registration patterns of the 117 women in the project to a group of 499 women who received prenatal care at one of the five participating sites, a local university-affiliated women's clinic (OU–TMC). This group was seen for prenatal care just before the special project was initiated and was judged to be roughly comparable to the project group in terms of education and income—perhaps slightly better off than the project group on both measures. The age distribution of the two groups was about the same, but the OU–TMC group had about half the proportion of black women that the project group did (16 percent versus 30 percent). Based on this difference, women in the OU–TMC group would be expected to register earlier in prenatal care than women in the patient advocate group. Nonetheless, 51 percent of the special intervention group registered for prenatal care in the first trimester, compared to 29 percent in the OU–TMC group. Among white women, the percentages were 51 versus 30; among black women, 47 versus 26; and among teenagers, 47 versus 28 percent.

Although self-selection issues and questions about the comparability of the groups loom large in this project, a reasonable conclusion is that this free pregnancy testing service coupled with social support probably contributed to earlier registration in prenatal care. Tulsa area officials share this generally positive view of the program and have provided for a year's continuation, although the program has been revised. For example, at present, paid staff have replaced volunteers as patient advocates.

The Special Supplemental Food Program for Women, Infants, and Children (WIC)—Six Studies

One of the objectives of the WIC program is to ensure that pregnant women receive adequate prenatal care. WIC agencies are required to check that pregnant women are obtaining care and to refer them if they are not; in a parallel effort, prenatal clinics often state that linking pregnant women to WIC services is one of their functions. Consequently, in communities where WIC is available, women might be expected to seek prenatal care earlier by virtue of close referral links. Similarly, women who obtain prenatal care at facilities that also house the WIC program might be expected to keep more of their prenatal appointments if the appointments were scheduled on the days they could obtain WIC vouchers. (A recent Department of Health and Human Services publication, *Improving MCH/ WIC Coordination*, provides numerous suggestions for improving the relationship between these two agencies; it also includes case reports of eight state programs.[24])

Several studies have explored the relationship between participation in WIC and use of prenatal care. The largest is Rush's historical study, which, beginning in 1972 with the Commodity Supplemented Food Program and extending through 1980, linked the proportion of eligible pregnant women served each year by the WIC program in individual counties ("WIC penetration") to levels of prenatal care for the same county and year.[25] A statistically significant relationship was found between WIC program penetration and both first-trimester registration and higher numbers of visits. The benefits were greatest among women with less education. Rush concluded that the WIC program is an inducement to and a vehicle for achieving greater use of prenatal care.

More recent studies have confirmed this conclusion. Among Massachusetts women who delivered in 1978, those who participated in WIC, as compared to a non-WIC group matched by age, race, parity, education, and marital status, had a higher number of prenatal visits (11.8 versus 10.8) and started care earlier (2.7 versus 2.9 months).[26] These results were all statistically significant, although they may not be programmatically meaningful. There was a large difference, however, in the percentage with inadequate care, as measured by the Kessner index (3.9 percent in the WIC group versus 7.0 percent in the non-WIC group).

Schramm conducted two studies of Missouri women who delivered in the early 1980s. The first study was of women enrolled in Medicaid who delivered in 1980.[27] In this analysis, with no variables controlled, women on WIC were less likely to have had inadequate prenatal care (defined by a combination of frequency of visits and number of weeks pregnant) than those not on WIC (39.1 percent versus 41.5 percent). In a 1982 replication, the percentage of WIC participants receiving inadequate prenatal care had been reduced to 35.4, while the percentage of non-WIC had increased to 44.8. Schramm suggested that the increased difference might reflect an improvement in referral patterns among WIC providers or changes in the types of mothers participating.[28]

Stockbauer also published two studies of Missouri births, but the analyses were not limited to women enrolled in Medicaid and were adjusted for race and education. In a study of 1980 births, the percentage of mothers obtaining inadequate prenatal care was higher in the WIC than in the non-WIC group (32.8 versus 29.5).[29] However, in a 1982 replication that controlled for a larger number of variables, the percentage receiving inadequate prenatal care was lower in the WIC group overall (30.4 percent versus 31.7 percent), significantly lower among blacks (32.1 percent versus 37.9 percent), but slightly higher among whites (29.5 percent versus 28.4 percent).[30]

Baby Showers—Seven Counties in Michigan[31]

The Detroit–Wayne County Infant Health Promotion Coalition not only organized the 961-BABY hotline described above, but also sponsored a series of community baby showers. These events were directed at identifying pregnant women early in pregnancy, enrolling them in a comprehensive prenatal care program, and sustaining their enrollment. They were also designed to identify women with infants in need of pediatric care and related social services.

In essence, the showers were casefinding and health education sessions that were open to the public and that included prepared presentations, small group discussions, and opportunities to make appointments on the spot for selected maternity, pediatric, and social services. In addition, various gifts, door prizes, and other incentives were offered throughout the day in order to create a baby shower atmosphere, encourage attendance, and underline the health education messages. In each county, the showers were publicized in advance by such efforts as door-to-door canvassing, direct mailings, posters, public health nurses' spreading the word, local McDonalds and grocery stores handing out shower invitations, billboards, car signs, "Mother's Day" sermons in target area churches, school presentations, and poster contests.

Eight showers were given in seven counties from October to December 1985. Attendance at the baby showers varied from 287 in Detroit to 34 in one county, for a total of 689. Approximately half the participants were black and more than a third were teenagers. Almost 70 percent of attendees were pregnant (478), but only 3 percent (21 women) were not receiving prenatal care already. Nonetheless, 74 prenatal appointments were made at the baby showers—a few for the women not in care, but most for those who stated they were already in care but who, in the opinion of the shower sponsors, required additional supervision. An additional 148 appointments were made for a variety of other services, including pediatric care, WIC, family planning, and social services. No information is available on the percentage of appointments actually kept.

Although the showers may have provided health education and social support, as well as facilitating the use of some services, their value as a casefinding tool for pregnant women not already in care was clearly limited. Anecdotal reports from similar efforts in California suggest greater casefinding success from this type of activity. The director estimates that the eight showers cost about $32,000 in the aggregate, not counting the substantial in-kind contributions of the sponsoring agencies and volunteers.

One major value of the showers may be that they increased the involvement of various church and community groups in issues of infant mortality and maternal health. This consciousness-raising function for the middle-class organizers of the events included a new appreciation of the problems faced by low-income women in securing prenatal and pediatric health care.

Type 5: Programs That Provide Social Support

Many projects offering intense social support to improve pregnancy outcome have been implemented in recent years. In this section, several are described beginning with the Resource Mothers Program in South Carolina, which focuses exclusively on adolescents. Following this is a summary of six additional comprehensive programs for pregnant adolescents. The section concludes with a description of the Prenatal and Infancy Home Visiting Program in Elmira, New York, and a brief note on the Grannies Program in Bibb County, Georgia.

Resource Mothers—Three Counties in South Carolina[32]

The Resource Mothers (RM) Program began in 1981 as a component of the Robert Wood Johnson Foundation's Rural Infant Care Program. It was originally confined to a three-county area, the Pee-Dee, which is very poor and rural, with few adequate health facilities and a postneonatal mortality rate (deaths that occur between 28 days and 12 months of age) in 1980 that was the highest of all 200 Health Service Areas in the United States.

The RM Program is for teenagers under 18 who are pregnant with their first child. The project emphasizes social support, health education and information, and general assistance offered by a Resource Mother. Teenagers are referred to the program by schools, health departments, private physicians, service agencies, civic and church groups, and peers. The Resource Mothers themselves are all mothers (many were pregnant as teenagers), high school graduates, and residents of the target counties. According to the project director, they are chosen on the basis of "personal warmth, successful personal parenting experiences, knowledge of community resources, demonstrated ability to accept responsibility, evidence of natural leadership, ability to use written and spoken language effectively, and subtle interpersonal skills." Resource Mothers participate in a 6-week training course. In addition, there are biweekly continuing education sessions and patient reviews with a social worker supervisor. The average caseload for a Resource Mother is 30 to 35 pregnant and postpartum teenagers.

Resource Mothers visit the participating teenagers at home or in other settings during pregnancy, in the hospital at the time of delivery, and during the first year postpartum. Visits are scheduled more often if there is a crisis. Although the visits are very structured, with a well-defined approach and specific content to be covered at each session, the Resource Mothers are encouraged to get to know the girl and her family very well—to become involved. They make sure that appointments are kept, providing transportation if necessary, and that recommendations from physicians and others are followed.

The program has been the subject of several evaluations, many of them focusing on reductions in low birthweight and improvements in infant development, since those are major goals of the program. The Committee, however, reviewed only those studies that examined use of prenatal care. One retrospective analysis compared a sample of RM women with matched controls drawn from the *same* counties. Women in both groups had a first, live birth (single) during the 1981–1985 interval. Using birth certificate records, controls were selected from women under 19 who had no known previous pregnancy; matching variables were year of delivery, county of residence, and race and sex of the child. Adequate controls were found for 519 of 575 RM cases. Of the RM clients, 17.5 percent evidenced inadequate prenatal care (fewer than five visits or care begun after the sixth month of pregnancy) versus 24.5 percent of the controls; the RM women averaged 8.6 prenatal visits versus 7.9 for the controls.[33]

Because of concern that selection bias limited the validity of these observed differences, a second retrospective analysis was conducted in which the controls were drawn from *different* counties that were nonetheless sociodemographically comparable to the Pee Dee area in which the RM Program operated. The study matched 565 women who had participated in the RM Program between 1981 and 1985 with women from nearby rural counties who also had first, live births (single) and no previous pregnancies; variables matched were year of delivery, maternal age, and child's race and sex. Of RM patients, 18.3 percent had received inadequate prenatal care versus 35.9 percent of the controls.[34]

The program still operates in the Pee Dee and has been expanded to other areas of the state as well. At present, some 16 Resource Mothers are at work in 20 counties, financed primarily by federal funds. Although state funds have been sought, few have been provided. Program leaders claim that state officials seem favorably impressed by the project, but thus far competing demands for public dollars have been too strong to allow RM much state support.[33]

Comprehensive Service Programs for Pregnant Adolescents— A Summary of Six Programs[35,36]

Because the needs of pregnant adolescents are so great, many communities have developed comprehensive programs to meet them. Such programs usually include, at a minimum, educational, social, and medical services in one facility or by referral. These types of programs have been encouraged and sometimes funded by the federal Office of Adolescent Pregnancy Programs. As with most of the services described in this appendix, few comprehensive adolescent programs use only one method to draw teenagers into prenatal care and sustain their participation. The three most commonly employed by the six programs described in this section are improving institutional arrangements, casefinding, and social support. The six projects summarized are the

Teen Mother and Child Program at the University of Utah School of Medicine; Youth Health Services in Elkins, West Virginia; the Teenage Pregnancy and Parenting Project in San Francisco; the adolescent program of the Visiting Nurse Association of Manchester and Southern New Hampshire; the Ethnic Adolescent Family Life Project in Providence, Rhode Island; and Johns Hopkins Hospital's Adolescent Pregnancy Program in Baltimore.

Improving Institutional Arrangements Adolescents frequently have difficulty using health services designed for older women. Hours may conflict with school, the site may be difficult to reach without a car, education may be minimal, and provider attitudes may be negative. All of the six programs address such issues by holding separate clinic sessions for teenagers, emphasizing continuity of providers, holding special group educational sessions, and so on. Some programs use vans to pick up clients at home and take them to sessions. A program serving rural adolescents provides transportation to and from the program site, the prenatal clinic, the WIC office, and other agencies. An inner-city program has developed a prenatal clinic in a school, providing medical care, prenatal education classes, and counseling and referral. Two programs have nurse–practitioners providing routine prenatal care because of their special skills in working with this age group. Other programs use nurse–practitioners for educational sessions and support during labor. One program provides in-home nursing care to adolescents between medical appointments. The visiting nurses provide routine health assessments, counseling, and prenatal and parenting education.

Casefinding Programs for adolescents rely heavily on referrals from current and former clients. Clients are educated to the need for such referrals. In one program, if an adolescent is missed—that is, not identified at an appropriate time—the staff asks currently enrolled clients how they could have found her earlier. Schools are an obvious source of referrals for adolescents. One program stations workers in two inner-city high schools 1 day a week. Students who have been identified as pregnant by a teacher or school nurse or who are suspected of being pregnant are seen by the worker during school time and helped to register for care. Pregnancy testing sites are also used to locate pregnant adolescents. One program continually reminds private physicians of its presence in order to obtain referrals. Another has a counselor visit adolescents who have been referred but who have not made contact with the program.

Social Support Many programs assign each teenage participant to a single individual (one program calls her a "continuous counselor") who coordinates and integrates the many services typically required by pregnant teenagers. While such counselors have traditionally been social workers, they may also be nurses, nutritionists, or other staff members. One program director said, "We have to rid ourselves of the medical model in serving teens. Teens need to be treated as whole persons. We can't have one practitioner counseling them in the clinic and another going out to make home visits. Everybody does everything here." These case supervisors provide counseling, education, referrals, advocacy, and follow-up, addressing the entire constellation of client needs. They must be able to become a "significant other" for young women who lack support from family members; in some programs they are expected to be available during nonworking hours, visit homes in inner-city neighborhoods, and provide support during labor. Bilingual case supervisors are often recruited by programs serving linguistic minorities.

Evaluation   The six programs have all studied the results of their activities by comparing program participants to other, similar groups on various measures of pregnancy outcome and use of prenatal care; none, however, has used randomization to overcome the possibility of selection bias. Five of the six programs demonstrated earlier entry into prenatal care, more prenatal visits, or both in comparison to a control group of adolescents. Only one program (the Ethnic Adolescent Family Life Project) found that the special program group entered prenatal care later and had fewer visits than the comparison group.

The Prenatal and Infancy Home Visiting Program— Elmira, New York[37]

This research and demonstration project was carried out between 1978 and the early 1980s in the target community of Elmira, which is semirural and located in the Appalachian region. In 1980 its economic conditions were rated the worst of all U.S. Standard Metropolitan Statistical Areas; its rates of child abuse and neglect were the highest in the state; and its infant mortality rate during the 1975–1977 interval, prior to the study, was 15.2 per 1,000 live births.

The program was designed to prevent a wide range of health and developmental problems in children through prenatal and postpartum home visiting by nurses. A sophisticated research and evaluation plan was built into the program at the outset. Pregnant women were recruited into the program if they had no previous live births and one or more of the following additional risk characteristics: under 19 years old, single, and low socioeconomic status. Other women expecting their first babies who asked to participate were also admitted.

Four hundred women were enrolled, stratified by marital status, race, and geographical region within the county, and assigned at random to one of four groups: (T1) assessment of the infant but no services; (T2) services limited to infant assessment and transportation assistance; (T3) home visiting during pregnancy only, plus transportation assistance and infant assessment; and (T4) same as (T3), but visiting continued through the first 2 years of the child's life. Nurses visited families about once every 2 weeks during the pregnancy, for an average of nine visits, each of which lasted over an hour. The visits had three basic objectives: parent education, the enhancement of women's informal support systems, and the linkage of women with community services. The nurses were taught to emphasize the strengths of the women and their families. (In assessing program results, the few nonwhite women in the program and women with maternal or fetal conditions that might lead to preterm birth were eliminated from the analyses.)

There was no difference between the groups visited by nurses (T3 and T4) and those not (T1 and T2) in number of prenatal care visits made by the pregnant women: both sets averaged about 10.5 visits, reflecting in part the fact that prenatal services were easily available through nine area obstetricians and a free antepartum clinic sponsored by the health department. There were, however, differences between the groups visited by nurses and those not visited on several other prenatal factors. For example, the visited women were aware of more community services, attended childbirth classes more frequently, received more WIC vouchers, talked more with service providers and members of their informal networks about the stresses of pregnancy and family life, indicated that their babies' fathers showed a greater interest in their pregnancies, and were accompanied more frequently in labor. Smokers who were visited reduced their smoking more than those who were not. The program is still operating, but as the years proceed and staff change, its original clarity of purpose and energy have diminished. Supported at first with federal research dollars, it is now funded by state monies and administered through the local health department.

The Grannies Program—Bibb County, Georgia[38]

The Grannies Program provides social support via the telephone. Women who come to the Bibb County health department prenatal clinic are assigned a Granny, who calls them twice a month before their babies are born and once a month for 12 months afterward. Grannies are paid by the hour and work out of their homes. They are supervised by a part-time program coordinator. The Grannies remind patients of their clinic appointments, suggest ways to obtain assistance when needed, and provide education and support.

The rate of broken appointments at the clinic has fallen from about 34 percent to 10 percent since the program has been in operation. Other measures of impact, such as trimester of registration, are not available.

REFERENCES AND NOTES

1. Descriptive material and data provided by the Division of Family Health Services, Massachusetts Department of Public Health; Katherine Messenger and Hannah Boulton, Massachusetts Department of Public Health. Personal communication, 1987–1988.
2. Azzara CV, Kotelchuch M, Anderka MT, Clark KS, and Robanske D. A Preliminary Healthy Start Evaluation: Interim Report for the Massachusetts Legislature. Boston: Division of Family Health Services, Department of Public Health, March 1988.
3. Descriptive material and data provided by the Michigan Department of Public Health; Janet Olszewski, Michigan Department of Public Health. Personal communication, 1988.
4. Maternal and Child Health Branch. Final Evaluation of the Obstetrical Access Pilot Project, July 1979–June 1982. Sacramento: California Department of Health Services, 1984; Korenbrot CC. Risk reduction in pregnancies of low-income women: Comprehensive prenatal care through the OB Access Project. Mobius 4:34–43, 1984; Lennie JA, Klun JR, and Hausner T. Low-birthweight rate reduced by the Obstetrical Access Project. Health Care Financing Rev. 8:83–86, 1987; Athole Lennie and Lyn Headley, California Department of Health Services. Personal communication, 1987–1988
5. Berger LR. Public/private cooperation in rural maternal child health efforts: The Lea county perinatal program. Tex. Med. 80:54–57, September 1984; Canfield E. The Select Panel Report—a follow-up. Paper presented at the American Public Health Association annual meeting, Los Angeles, 1981; Russell RE. The first report on the Lea County survey of women who have delivered babies while residents of Lea County during 1976–1981. Unpublished paper, 1982; Spice B. Program reduces infant death rate. Albuquerque Joual, January 5, 1987; Lawrence Berger, Lovelace Medical Foundation. Personal communication, 1987–1988.
6. Description of Prenatal Care Assistance Program, New York State Department of Health, December 30, 1987; PCAP client characteristics, services, and pregnancy outcomes, New York State Department of Health, September 21, 1987; Linda Randolph, New York State Department of Health. Personal communication, 1987–1988.
7. Division of Maternal–Fetal Medicine, State University of New York and Onondaga County Health Department. Prevention of low birthweight program in Onondaga County. Proposal for funding to Department of Health, State of New York, 1983; Richard Aubry, Health Science Center, State University of New York. Personal communication, 1987–1988.
8. Sokol RJ, Wolf RB, Rosen MG, and Weingarden K. Risk, antepartum care, and outcome: Impact of a Maternity and Infant Care Project. Obstet. Gynecol. 56:150–156, 1980; Elizabeth Campbell, Cleveland Metropolitan General Hospital. Personal communication, 1987.
9. Peoples MD and Siegel E. Measuring the impact of programs for mothers and infants on prenatal care and low birth weight: The value of refined analysis. Med. Care 21:586–605, 1983.

10. Health Services Administration, Bureau of Community Health Services. The Maternity and Infant Care Projects: Reducing Risks for Mothers and Babies. DHEW Pub. No. (HSA)75-5012. Rockville, Md., 1975, p. 15.
11. Ibid., p. 16.
12. Peoples MD, Grimson RC, and Daughtry GL. Evaluation of the effects of the Carolina Improved Pregnancy Outcome Project: Implications for state-level decision making. Am. J. Public Health 74:549–554, 1984.
13. Strobino DM, Chase GA, Kim YJ, Crawley BE, Salim JH, and Baruffi G. The impact of the Mississippi improved child health project on prenatal care and low birthweight. Am. J. Public Health 76:274–278, 1986.
14. Jones JE, Tiezzi L, and Williams-Kaye J. Notes from the field: Overcoming barriers to Medicaid eligibility. Am. J. Public Health 76:1247, 1986; Jones JE, Tiezzi L, and Williams-Kaye J. Financial access: Key to early prenatal care. Paper presented at the American Public Health Association annual meeting, Washington, D.C., 1985; Judith Jones, National Resource Center for Children in Poverty, Columbia University. Personal communication, 1987–1988.
15. Rural infant deaths decline with aid of UT Memphis project. The Record (University of Tennessee Health Science Center), February 1987; Ryan GM. Papers presented at the Orange County Obstetric and Gynecological Congress, Costa Mesa, Calif., April 3, 1987, and at the Boston Obstetrical Society, March 23, 1981; George Ryan, Department of Obstetrics and Gynecology, University of Tennessee. Personal communication, 1987–1988.
16. Brooks-Gunn J, McCormick MC, Gunn RW, Shorter T, Wallace CY and Haegarty MC. Locating low-income pregnant women: The process of outreach. Medical Care, in press.; McCormick MC, Brooks-Gunn J, Shorter T, Holmes JH, Wallace CY, and Haegarty MC. Outreach as casefinding: Its effect on enrollment in prenatal care. Medical Care, in press; Margaret Haegarty, Harlem Hospital Center. Personal communication, 1987.
17. Jones J. Community health advocate program: Final report to The Ford Foundation, April 1981–September 1982; Judith Jones, National Resource Center for Children in Poverty, Columbia University. Personal communication, 1987–1988.
18. Deborah Coates and Joan Maxwell, The Better Babies Project. Personal communication, 1987–1988.
19. Christison-Lagay J. The maternity and infant outreach project of the Hartford Action Plan on Infant Health. Unpublished report, 1986; Joan Christison-Lagay, Hartford City Health Department. Personal communication, 1987–1988.
20. Breitbart V and Zeitel L. Hotline As a Means to Improve Access to Prenatal Care in New York City. New York: Bureau of Maternity Services and Family Planning, New York City Department of Health, 1986; Vicki Breithart, Bureau of Maternity Services and Family Planning, New York City Department of Health. Personal communication, 1987–1988.
21. Wright TD. Evaluation of 961-BABY: A telephone information and referral service. Paper presented at the American Public Health Association annual meeting, Las Vegas, 1986; Terri Wright, Detroit/Wayne County Infant Health Promotion Coalition. Personal communication, 1987.
22. CHOICE. Hotline data report July 1, 1985–June 30, 1986, submitted to the Philadelphia Department of Public Health; Muriel Keyes, CHOICE. Personal communication, 1987–1988.
23. Jackson CJ, Renner S and Lapolla M. The Use of Free Pregnancy Testing to Encourage Early Entry into Prenatal Care. Tulsa: Oklahoma Medical Research

Foundation, Center for Health Policy Research, 1987; Cassandra Jackson, Center for Health Policy Research. Personal communication, 1987–1988.

24. Improving MCH/WIC Coordination—Final Report and Guide to Good Practices. Submitted by Professional Management Associates, Inc. to the Office of the Assistant Secretary of Planning and Evaluation, Department of Health and Human Services. Contract No. HHS-100-84-0069, Washington, D.C., August 1986.

25. Rush D. Evaluation of the Special Supplemental Food Program for Women, Infants and Children (WIC). Vol. I: Summary. Submitted by Research Triangle Institute to the Office of Analysis and Evaluation, Food and Nutrition Service, Department of Agriculture. Contract No. 53-3198-9-87, Washington, D.C., January 1986.

26. Kotelchuck M, Schwartz JB, Anderka MT, and Finison KS. WIC participation and pregnancy outcomes: Massachusetts statewide evaluation project. Am. J. Public Health 74:1086–1092, 1984.

27. Schram WF. WIC participation and its relationship to newborn Medicaid costs in Missouri: A cost-benefit analysis. Am. J. Public Health 75:851–857, 1985.

28. Schram WF. Prenatal participation in WIC related to Medicaid costs for Mississippi newborns: 1982 update. Public Health Reps. 101:607–615, 1986.

29. Stockbauer JW. Evaluation of the Missouri WIC program: Prenatal component. J. Am. Dietet. Assoc. 86:61–67, 1986.

30. Stockbauer JW. WIC prenatal participation and its relation to pregnancy outcomes in Missouri: A second look. Am. J. Public Health 77:813–818, 1987.

31. Wright TD and O'Meara M. Community Baby Shower Summary Report: Regional Outreach Campaign, Fall 1985. Detriot: Detroit/Wayne County Infant Health Promotion Coalition, 1986; Terri Wright, Detroit/Wayne County Infant Health Promotion Coalition. Personal communication, 1987.

32. Lois Wandersman and Marie Meglen, South Carolina Department of Health and Environmental Control. Personal communication, 1987–1988.

33. Meglen MC and Wandersman LP. Perinatal impact of South Carolina's Resource Mothers Program. Unpublished paper, 1987.

34. Heins HC, Nance NW, and Ferguson JE. Social support in improving perinatal outcome: The Resource Mothers Program. Obstet. Gynecol. 70:263–266, 1987.

35. Cartoof VG. Increasing adolescents' access to prenatal care: A case study of six programs. Paper prepared for the Committee on Outreach for Prenatal Care, Institute of Medicine, Washington, D.C. 1987.

36. Elster AB, Lamb ME, Tavare J, and Ralston CW. The medical and psychosocial impact of comprehensive care on adolescent pregnancy and parenthood. J. Am. Med. Assoc. 258:1187–1192, 1987.

37. Olds DL, Henderson CR, Tatelbaum, R and Chamberlin R. Improving the delivery of prenatal care and outcomes of pregnancy: A randomized trial of nurse home visitation. Pediatrics 77:16–28, 1986; David Olds, Department of Pediatrics, University of Rochester. Personal communication, 1988.

38. Jacqueline Scott, Bibb County Health Department. Personal communication, 1987.

Appendix

B

Prenatal Care Outreach: An International Perspective

C. Arden Miller

Infant mortality rates are generally lower in Western Europe than in the United States, a circumstance that has attracted comment from health policy analysts for several decades. The trend during this time has been toward continued lowering of rates among all industrialized nations, yet the United States' relative rank has dropped (Children's Defense Fund, 1987). Recent adverse trends in several U.S. indicators of maternal and infant health (Miller et al., 1986; Children's Defense Fund, 1987) have sharpened interest in how countries with the lowest rates achieve them (National Center for Health Statistics, 1985b).

An opportunity to review perinatal supports, services, and financing in Europe came in 1982, with the completion of a 23-nation survey conducted by the Perinatal Study Group convened by the World Health Organization Regional Office for Europe (EURO). The 15-member group represented 10 countries and 10 different professional disciplines (economics, epidemiology, health administration, midwifery, nursing, obstetrics, pediatrics, psychology, sociology, and statistics). The results of the survey were summarized in two works (Regional Office for Europe, 1985;

This paper is condensed from a larger work, entitled *Perinatal Care in Europe: Implications for U.S. Policy*, published by the National Center for Clinical Infant Programs, Washington, D.C., 1987. The work was supported by a Fulbright Grant and the Ford Foundation, and was facilitated by Marsden Wagner, Regional Officer for Maternal and Child Health, World Health Organization, Regional Office for Europe, Copenhagen. C. Arden Miller is Professor, Department of Maternal and Child Health, School of Public Health, University of North Carolina, Chapel Hill.

Phaff, 1986). Although the information is useful and important, much of it is descriptive and cannot be linked to individual countries. Identification of models that might be of special interest in U.S. policy formulation is clouded by the aggregation of survey findings among countries with diverse social and political traditions and with a wide range of accomplishment in perinatal care.

In 1986, Marsden Wagner, Regional Officer for Maternal and Child Health for EURO, granted me permission to review the raw responses to the 1982 survey. He also arranged for the national files at EURO to be opened for inspection and made available the proofs of the World Health Organization's (WHO's) seventh annual report on the world health situation (World Health Organization, 1986). That work contains WHO's most recent statistical tabulations of health status for each country as well as narratives on the health care system of each. Other useful sources of information are the periodic reports from UNICEF (1987) and the World Bank (1986). In addition, I visited academics, health officials, researchers, and clinic providers in Denmark, Federal Republic of Germany, Netherlands, Belgium, and the United Kingdom. Experts from each of these countries were asked to review the ensuing report, and I have incorporated their suggestions for revision. These advisers were especially helpful in directing my attention to reports on relevant research in Europe. Although extensive writings on perinatal care in Western Europe were reviewed, their scope does not embrace the full range of available literature—and none of the literature printed in languages other than English.

STUDY COUNTRIES

The Perinatal Study Group characterized each country's health care system as monopolistic, pluralistic, or intermediate, and categorized survey responses accordingly. Monopolistic systems of health care were identified as those in which " . . . pregnancy and birth care is offered exclusively through institutions such as health centers and maternity outpatient and inpatient departments. In these institutions all personnel are employed by the state" (Regional Office for Europe, 1985, pp. 7–8). In pluralistic systems, " . . . care during pregnancy and birth is provided by midwives and doctors in private practice and, to a lesser extent, through institutions. The woman is relatively free to choose the type of care she wants" (Regional Office for Europe, 1985, p. 8). Intermediate systems have features of both.

Countries that were characterized as having monopolistic systems of health care were excluded from this analysis because their experience is unlikely to have much relevance for U.S. policy. On this basis Finland and

Sweden were excluded, even though both have an outstanding record of maternity care and are frequently cited in international comparisons of maternal and child health services (Wallace, 1975; National Center for Health Statistics, 1985a). Nearly all prenatal care in these countries is rendered in public clinics, and women must deliver in a hospital that is determined by place of residence, circumstances that are not likely to come about in the United States.

Designation of the United Kingdom's system as an intermediate one deserves comment. Although the National Health Service has been in operation since 1948, pregnant women may choose place of delivery, a small private sector of physician providers persists, and private health insurance coverage is growing in importance. In addition, the physician providers, although they contract with the National Health Service, are not government employees.

Inclusion of Spain and Ireland in the study group is noteworthy because they are less affluent than the other nations in the study. Both have undertaken important health service reforms in recent years and have achieved impressive new records for infant survival. Countries with populations of less than one million and countries with infant mortality rates higher than that of the United States were also excluded. Ten countries remained for analysis (see Table 1).

TABLE 1   Rates of Infant Mortality and Low Birthweight in the Study Countries, 1982[a]

Country	Infant Mortality Rate[b]	Low Birthweight Rate[c]
Belgium	10.10	5
Denmark	7.71	6[d]
France	9.40	5
Federal Republic of Germany	10.20	5
Ireland	10.10	4
Netherlands	8.40	4
Norway	7.90	4
Spain	9.60	NA
Switzerland	7.60	5
United Kingdom	10.00	7

[a]The infant mortality rate is the number of deaths per 1,000 births. The low birthweight rate is the number of newborns weighing 2,500 grams or less per 1,000 live births. Data are usually for 1982.
[b]World Health Organization, 1986.
[c]UNICEF, 1987.
[d]Other sources report a rate of four for Denmark (World Health Organization, 1986).

ADEQUACY OF DATA

Research on prenatal care in the United States focuses on timing—the stage of pregnancy at which the first visit occurs and the number of subsequent visits—because those data are readily available on birth certificates. Scant data are available on the content of prenatal visits (Institute of Medicine, 1985). Insofar as criteria for the adequacy of care have been developed, they are framed in terms of the number of visits in the various stages of pregnancy (Kessner, 1973). Cost and cost-effectiveness attract attention (Institute of Medicine, 1985).

Comparable data are not generally available for Europe. Data are available on the number of prenatal visits to various providers, but information on the timing of the first prenatal visit is conspicuously lacking. All advisers insist, without recourse to confirming data, that attracting women to the first prenatal visit is not a problem because many perinatal benefits are contingent on confirming the pregnancy and registering it with the appropriate official agencies, tasks undertaken at the first visit. The focus in improving prenatal care is on women who do not return after the first visit. Blondel (1987) reports that in the study countries less than 2 percent of women who deliver have had no prenatal care.

Standards of perinatal care are established for all countries and are expressed in terms of entitlement to health services and social supports. The number of visits, examinations, laboratory tests, screening procedures, home visits, income transfers, and other benefits are specified for every country. In some countries (for example, Norway), the number and content of prenatal visits take the form of government-sanctioned recommendations rather than legal regulations. The survey inquired about the existence of national standards and asked for certain particulars about them. A full reporting of standards was not requested and was usually not provided.

The EURO survey inquired about the use of prenatal screening procedures (blood testing, toxoplasmosis, rubella, tetanus, syphilis, amniocentesis, and ultrasound), and those results have been reported (Regional Office for Europe, 1985).

A study committee working on behalf of the European Economic Community has conducted a survey of teaching hospitals on the recommended content of prenatal visits. Complete results are not yet available, but variation among nations is said to be exceedingly great (P. Buekens, personal communication, 1986). For example, in France and Germany the cervix is routinely examined during prenatal visits; in the United Kingdom (and the United States) such examinations are done only for special indications. The pros and cons of these two approaches have not been evaluated.

Adequate data on the cost of prenatal care and its various components are not available. Even when the aggregate costs of the entire perinatal sequence are reported, comparisons are suspect; some reports appear to include income supplements that are associated with childbearing, whereas others appear to confine themselves to medical costs.

To the extent that data are available on cost, they focus on the use of hospitals. Many countries have attempted to reduce hospital expenses by relying on home care and outpatient visits. These strategies are considered to be less expensive than hospital care, but careful cost-benefit analyses are not generally available. An exception is the Netherlands, where the expense of the extensive postnatal home visiting program has come under review. That review appears to ask only about the possible disadvantages that might result if home visiting, lasting up to 8 hours a day for 10 days (averaging 64 hours for every delivery in 1986), were reduced to 7 days. Several reports emphasize that either home care or outpatient care is less expensive than keeping new mothers and their babies in the hospital more than 36 hours after birth (in the absence of medical indications to the contrary).

Responses to the survey were enormously instructive but diverse in style. Some queries that asked for data were completed with a narrative. Others that requested a narrative were answered with a word or a copy of a multipage published report. In the analysis that follows, I have attempted to adhere to a quantitative treatment, but descriptions and undocumented generalizations are given when they contribute to an understanding of well-established practice as represented in the survey responses.

Research and precise documentation of perinatal care in Europe are actively pursued but, understandably, not with the same urgency as in the United States.

CHARACTERISTICS OF STUDY COUNTRIES

Several factors affecting prenatal care in the 10 study countries deserve consideration.

Demographics

Comparisons of the human services offered in the United States and in European countries are sometimes discounted on the basis of the belief that the heterogeneity of the U.S. population complicates delivery of care more here than in Europe. That reasoning is weakened if one regards the considerable migration into Western Europe since World War II of persons from the Middle East, North Africa, and various former colonies.

For example, foreign-born persons make up 10.6 percent of the population of France, 16.7 percent of Switzerland, and 8.8 percent of the United Kingdom (Demographic Yearbook, 1983). Proportions are much higher in some cities. In Amsterdam, 18.2 percent of the population is foreign-born (Doornbos and Nordbeck, 1985), and the proportion for Brussels was 23.9 percent in 1981 (Buekens, personal communicaton, 1986). The large contribution of nonindigenous populations to the problems of childbearing is most strikingly revealed by data on the country of origin of children under five in Amsterdam in 1981: 44.5 percent were born to nonindigenous families, most commonly Surinamese or Moroccan (Doornbos and Nordbeck, 1985).

Many reports (Blondel et al., 1985; Doornbos and Norbeck, 1985; Kaminski et al., 1987) indicate that pregnancy-related use of services and outcomes of pregnancy are less favorable for immigrant women than for indigenous women, but the gaps are neither great nor consistent. In Amsterdam, 70 percent of Dutch women and 50 percent of immigrant women went for prenatal care within the first 16 weeks of pregnancy; subsequently, the immigrant women made more frequent visits. In Munich, women of non-Germanic origin (about 20 percent of deliveries) used public health services at the same rate as German women (Doornbos and Nordbeck, 1985). The quality of prenatal care for each of several national subgroups was judged to be similar for all patients delivered of babies at a large London hospital (cited by Buekens, 1987). Both in Amsterdam and in Munich, outcomes of pregnancy were less favorable for immigrant women. A letter from Buekens (1987) presents similar findings for Belgium in 1983, citing a perinatal mortality rate of 10.7 for Belgium women and higher rates for foreign-born women living in Belgium (Turkish, 17.8; North African, 14.8).

Not all studies demonstrate such a difference. In Sweden (not included among the study countries) non-Nordic immigrant families were shown to use health services extensively and to have pregnancy outcomes that were comparable to, if not more favorable than, those of Swedes (Smedby and Ericson, 1979). Doornbos and Nordbeck (1985) cite a study in West Germany demonstrating that perinatal mortality rates among Turkish immigrants were similar to those among the German population of the same socioeconomic status.

These data are not presented with the intent of establishing that circumstances for immigrant families in Europe are in every way parallel to those for indigenous minority families in the United States. Almost certainly a different set of problems pertains, but both situations involve overcoming barriers associated with sociocultural differences. Some special measures have been taken in Europe to overcome these differences; in the Netherlands, for example, health care providers and their patients who encounter a language barrier can obtain instantaneous, on-site translations over the telephone. None of the survey responses or other descriptions identified well-organized educational campaigns or other outreach efforts specifically directed toward immigrants.

All countries in the study except for the United Kingdom have lower rates of low birthweight than the United States (Table 1). When the U.S. rates are disaggregated by race, the rate for whites (5.6) is still substantially higher than the lowest European rates (4.0) (National Center for Health Statistics, 1987). These differences cannot be explained entirely on the basis of different rates of teenage childbearing. When corrections are made for other known variables, the contribution of maternal age to low birthweight is small (Institute of Medicine, 1985).

Population density is high in most of the countries, but the exceptions are important. Norway's population is widely scattered among many isolated communities. The average number of prenatal visits varies between 10 and 14 in all parts of the country. Pregnant women who live in remote areas are reimbursed for travel expenses and subsistence for 10 days in order to be near a hospital when delivery is expected.

The urban population of the study countries ranges from a low of 57 percent for Ireland to a high of 96 percent for Belgium. Four countries (France, Norway, Ireland, and Switzerland) have a less urbanized population than the United States (UNICEF, 1987).

Teenage Childbearing

The most important demographic difference between the United States and the 10 European nations is the age-specific fertility rate. Rates of teenage pregnancy, abortion, and childbearing are substantially lower in Europe (Jones et al., 1985). The rate of childbearing among 15- to 19-year-olds in the 1980s was roughly three times higher in the United States than in European countries (Table 2). That difference holds for both black and white populations, and it would be even greater if abortion did not interrupt nearly half the teenage pregnancies in the United States. This entire issue and its implications for infant survival have been carefully reviewed at the Alan Guttmacher Institute (Jones et al., 1985). Findings suggest that the age of onset of sexual activity does not vary greatly among these countries, but access to contraception is more limited and fewer children participate in organized programs of sex education in the United States.

A dramatic decline in rates of teenage childbearing in Europe took place during the 1970s, while the U.S. rate remained high (Table 2). That decline occurred in the context of extensively expanded medical and social benefits for pregnant women, including income supplements to help with

TABLE 2 Rate of Teenage Childbearing[a] in the United States and the Study Countries

Country	1970s	1980s
Belgium	31	19
Denmark	32	11
France	27	15
Federal Republic of Germany	36	10
Ireland	16	18
Netherlands	23	7
Norway	45	20
Spain	22	27[b]
Switzerland	22	8
United Kingdom	41	28
United States	64[c,d]	54[c]

[a]Live births per 1,000 women age 15–19.
[b]Data for 1979.
[c]Demographic Yearbook, 1973 and 1983.
[d]Data for 1969.

SOURCE: EURO files, 1986.

the expense of child rearing. Clearly, the expanded benefits did not induce teenagers to increase their fertility.

Household Income

The per-capita gross national product (GNP) in the United States and in Western Europe is high, but income alone does not account for low rates of infant mortality. A threefold difference in per capita GNP separates the European countries with the lowest values from those with the highest (Ireland and Spain with values of $5,230 and $5,640, respectively, and Switzerland with $17,430). Household income in the United States is higher than that in six study nations with better records of infant survival (World Health Organization, 1986).

The distribution of proportional shares of household income between the highest and lowest quintiles is interesting (Table 3). The gap between rich and poor is greater in the United States than in any other country except France, for which recent data are not available.

Redistribution of household income to reduce poverty might bring about many benefits, including a reduction in infant mortality rates. But the record clearly indicates that household wealth far below the U.S. average and income distributions nearly as disparate as those in the United States (in France, Denmark, and Spain, for example) are compatible with highly favorable rates of infant survival. Without in any way minimizing the urgency of lowering poverty rates, especially in households with children, one can make a compelling case that selective, direct approaches for improving outcomes of pregnancy are feasible within the present income structure of the United States. The recent records in Ireland and Spain are especially compelling in this regard. Barcelona, known to have extensive barrios of poverty and congestion, has an infant mortality rate of eight (EURO files, 1986).

National Finances

No country in the study spends as high a proportion of its GNP on health care as the United States (10.7 percent). Countries that emphasize insurance systems to reimburse private physician providers on a fee-for-service basis tend to spend more (Belgium, 9.1 percent; France, 8.0; Federal Republic of Germany, 9.3; Switzerland, 7.1) than countries that compensate providers at a negotiated, fixed per-capita rate (Denmark, 5.5 percent; United Kingdom, 6.1; Norway, 7.1; Netherlands, 8.8) or those that make extensive use of public clinics (Spain, 4.3 percent; Ireland, 7.4; and, in some areas, the United Kingdom and Norway) (World Health Organization, 1986).

The predominant health care provider systems and their means of financing vary greatly among the European countries, but they have been consistent in pursuing vigorously policies to reduce hospitalization other than for childbearing (World Health Organization, 1986). They have also

TABLE 3   Difference Between Highest and Lowest Quintiles in Proportional Share of Total Household Income in the United States and the Study Countries, 1979–1982

Country	Difference
Belgium	26.1
Netherlands	27.9
Switzerland	31.4
Federal Republic of Germany	31.6
Ireland (1973)	32.2
Norway	32.2
United Kingdom	32.7
Spain	33.1
Denmark	33.2
United States	34.6
France (1975)	40.3

SOURCE: Adapted from World Health Organization, 1986.

emphasized organized community services with decentralized administrations and uniform national standards for preventive measures. Increasing responsibility for health services has been placed on local governmental jurisdictions as the role of central government has been strengthened for standard setting, monitoring, and overall financing. Even in Switzerland, probably the most privatized system of health care among the 10 study countries, national standards for perinatal service are defined and their implementation subsidized by government grants to the insurance companies.

Health Care Financing and Delivery

Financing systems for health care are strikingly different among the countries and bear no consistent relationship to differences in prevailing health care provider systems. Insurance and social security schemes predominate, premium payments being made both by employers and by workers, as wage deductions. Insurance may be government run or controlled (Netherlands, Spain, Belgium), predominantly private (Switzerland), or a combination of public and private (Federal Republic of Germany, France). In four countries, all of which rely predominantly on office-based practitioners for primary care, financing comes entirely or in large part from general tax revenues (Denmark, United Kingdom, Ireland, Norway).

This diversity should not obscure a theme common to all the countries. No matter what the financing system, even when private intermediaries participate extensively, the central government has defined the services that are to be provided and, in the case of maternity care, has removed all barriers to those services. The full range of perinatal services is provided without charge to women of all socioeconomic levels, with only a few minor fees that are readily waived in the event of need.

MATERNITY-RELATED SERVICES

The survey inquired about public education programs and the use of communications media to inform women about the desirability and availability of prenatal care. Survey responses for all countries indicated that such activities go on, often under the auspices of volunteer organizations or public interest professional groups. The activities are described as occasional, random, and not aggressively organized. On the other hand, several reports emphasize the highly organized programs of education about sexuality and human reproduction that are conducted in European schools (Jones et al., 1985). Presumably those programs incorporate instruction about the importance of prenatal care, but that assumption was not investigated.

In several countries (Belgium, France, Federal Republic of Germany, Norway, and Switzerland) the usual procedure is for a pregnant woman to seek prenatal care from the general practitioner or obstetrician of her choice. In Denmark and the United Kingdom every person is registered with a general practitioner who serves as a gatekeeper to other services. In the United Kingdom that practitioner ordinarily continues prenatal care for uncomplicated pregnancies, arranging for a visit with the midwife and consultations, as needed, with obstetricians at the hospital where the woman is booked for delivery. In Denmark a precise schedule is followed, including two visits to an obstetrician, five to a midwife (who is a public employee), and three to the general practitioner. Public clinics are an option for care in Norway.

In the Netherlands a woman first sees a general practitioner and then decides to continue that care or be transferred to a privately practicing midwife, who would also deliver the baby. An obstetrician is seen only for complicated pregnancies. In Ireland and Spain women may seek care from an obstetrician or general practitioner of their choice, but recently emphasis has been placed on the use of multidisciplinary primary care public clinics. The general practitioner's role has declined except as a participant in those clinics. Specialists, such as obstetricians, are generally hospital-based and render their consultations in hospital outpatient departments.

Midwives are extensively involved in European maternity care. Their work is ordinarily confined to hospitals and multidisciplinary clinics except in the Netherlands, where they are independent, office-based practitioners. In Denmark midwives are government employees and work out of public offices or clinics; they participate in a schedule of routine prenatal care that includes visits to a general practitioner and to an obstetrician. A 1984 government report in Norway recommends 12 prenatal visits for uncomplicated pregnancies, half of them to a midwife and half to a general practitioner. In most countries, midwives attend uncomplicated deliveries for women who have received routine prenatal care from office-based general practitioners.

Public Clinics

Public clinics are sometimes regarded as an alternative to office-based physician practice. In Norway, for example, each municipality is required to maintain at least one public, multidisciplinary health center, even though care by office-based medical practitioners may be readily available. Multidisciplinary public clinics have been developed in selected locales of other countries to enhance services for hard-to-reach populations (Belgium, United Kingdom). Several countries have either phased out public clinics or have elected not to develop them, in the belief that access to physicians' offices is both assured and universally utilized (Denmark, Netherlands, Federal Republic of Germany, Switzerland, and France). Only two countries in the study (Ireland and Spain) have dramatically increased the number of public clinics recently, relying on them to provide multidisciplinary primary medical care (including perinatal care) and a number of social support services. Both of these countries were faced with the need to improve health conditions without major increase in expenditures, and in both countries these goals have been impressively realized.

Number of Prenatal Visits

The officially required or recommended number of prenatal visits for an uncomplicated pregnancy varies enormously (4 to 12). The average number of visits actually made closely approximates or exceeds the recommendations (Table 4). The survey responses did not provide data on the range of visits from which the averages were calculated.

The survey inquired about instructional classes for pregnant women. Many volunteer organizations, agencies, and clinics offer such classes, and they are reported to be well utilized, but they are not regularly institutionalized into standards of prenatal care.

TABLE 4   Prenatal Visits in the Study Countries, 1981–1982

Country	Number Recommended or Legally Required	Average Actual Number
Belgium (French-speaking sector)	7	9.4[a]
Denmark	10	8
Federal Republic of Germany	10	ND
France	7	5.9
Ireland	6	10 urban
		5 rural
Netherlands	12	12–14
Norway	12–14	>10 (39% of women)
Spain[b]	10	6
Switzerland	3–4	5
United Kingdom	12–13	10–12 (Scotland)

[a]Vandenbussche et al., 1985. Some characteristics of antenatal care in 13 European countries. Brit. J. Obstet. Gynaecol. 92:1297.

[b]I. Alvarez, personal communication, 1987.

SOURCE: EURO survey, 1982, adapted from Blondel, B., 1987.

Home Visiting

Home visiting is a feature of nearly every country's maternity care and is practiced more consistently after delivery than before (Table 5). For uncomplicated pregnancies, prenatal home visiting is extensively used to inquire about missed appointments in an effort to resolve any contributing problems. Home visitors are sometimes midwives, but they are more often nurses with special training for home visiting. No country makes use of health aides or neighborhood workers as home visitors except possibly the Netherlands, where an extensive postnatal homemaking service supplements routine postnatal visits by the midwife or general practitioner who rendered prenatal care.

TABLE 5 Home Visiting in the Study Countries, 1982[a]

PRENATAL VISITS
Always at least once
  Belgium (unevenly implemented)
  Denmark (unevenly implemented)
  Netherlands
Only for complicated pregnancies or to check on clinic nonattenders
  Belgium
  Federal Republic of Germany (not an extensive program)
  France
  Ireland[b]
  Norway
  Switzerland
  United Kingdom[b]

POSTNATAL VISITS
Always at least once
  Belgium
  Denmark
  Ireland
  Netherlands (daily visits for up to 8 hours through tenth day postpartum)
  Norway
  Switzerland
  United Kingdom (daily visits by a midwife or health visitor for 10 days)
Only for special indications
  Federal Republic of Germany
  France

[a]Spain is currently implementing a program for prenatal and postnatal home visiting. Services are not yet widely available (I. Alvarez, personal communication, 1987).
[b]Well-developed program for nonattenders.

SOURCE: EURO survey, 1982.

Postnatal home visiting in the Netherlands is a central theme of maternity care. Every woman is visited at home by either the midwife or the general practitioner. In addition, a specially trained maternity home helper stays with the mother and infant for up to 8 hours a day until the tenth day after birth. The visitor helps with infant care, shopping, housekeeping, meal preparation, and care of older siblings. In 1986 each newborn and mother received an average of 64 hours of postnatal home visiting (H. P. Verbrugge, personal communication, 1987). For this service the family pays only a token fee.

In all countries, postnatal home visiting is seen as a means for counseling about infant care, for follow-up on the mother's health, for advice on family planning, for initial or follow-up neonatal screening procedures, and for setting up additional appointments for the infant and mother.

Incentives to Participate in Prenatal Care

In two countries (France and Federal Republic of Germany) financial benefits, payable at the time of delivery, have been withheld from women who did not make a specified number of prenatal visits. In West Germany this practice has been discontinued, and the benefits are now rendered without reference to prenatal visitation; only France continues the practice of offering a financial bonus for women who have made at least three prenatal visits. Prenatal attendance in France, particularly among Algerian immigrant women, improved markedly during the 1970s. Between 1972 and 1981 the proportion of pregnant women with fewer than four prenatal visits fell from 15.3 percent to 3.9 percent (Maxwell, 1984). The influence of financial incentives on this trend is problematic. Buekens has examined evidence that attempts to evaluate the effectiveness of financial incentives and found the evidence inconclusive (Buekens, 1987). The French system places incentives in an explicit context with some punitive implications.

Another way of considering incentives is to regard the full range of benefits and supports associated with childbearing as incentives to seek prenatal care. These include transportation, early booking for delivery at a location of the woman's choice, paid leave from employment, birthing bonus, family allowances, home visitors, preference in housing, and children's allowances to help with the costs of child rearing. All of these are powerful incentives to register the pregnancy and impending delivery with the appropriate agencies, procedures ordinarily accomplished at the first prenatal visit.

In all European countries in the study, the incentives for participating in prenatal care are strong and the barriers are virtually nonexistent. Rather than ask why pregnant women participate so early and so consistently, one might instead ask, Why wouldn't they?

TABLE 6   Home Deliveries as a Percentage of
All Deliveries in Study Countries, 1979–1982[a]

Country	Percent
Belgium (1984)	0.4
Denmark	0.5
Federal Republic of Germany	1.0
France	0.5
Netherlands	35.4
Spain[a]	0.5
United Kingdom	1.4

[a]Precise data are not available for other countries beyond notations that home deliveries are rare or uncommon.

[b]I. Alvarez, personal communication, 1987.

SOURCE: EURO survey, 1982.

Home Deliveries

The proportion of home deliveries has declined everywhere and remains high only in the Netherlands, where it represents officially supported policy (Table 6). The Dutch insurance system will not compensate for an obstetrician's services or for a hospital delivery without a specific medical indication from an authorized list. New perinatal guidelines in Denmark encourage home deliveries, and they are increasing in some parts of the country.

Hospital Deliveries

Precise data on the duration of hospital stays for childbearing were not available. Evidence suggests that stays are longer in Europe than in the United States and that, when the stay is less than 5 days, the postnatal home visits are increased in frequency and duration.

The Netherlands provides for deliveries that are neither fully hospital-based nor fully home-based. A polyclinic delivery allows a woman and her attending midwife to arrange for delivery on hospital premises, stay for up to 36 hours, and then return home for the usual pattern of home visiting. The delivery is not recorded as a hospital admission, and hospitals are not compensated on that basis. About one-third of the nation's deliveries conform to this pattern.

Caesarean sections are performed at consistently lower rates in Europe (5 to 13 percent in 1983) than in the United States, where in 1985 the rate was 23 percent (Placek, 1986; Notzon et al., 1987). The trend is upward in all countries.

Continuity of Care

Continuity of care in the sense that one provider attends the same patient throughout the prenatal, intrapartum, and postnatal periods is not a prominent feature in any of the countries. Because a pregnant woman may receive prenatal care in more than one setting (practitioner's office and specialist's clinic at the hospital), be delivered by yet another provider (hospital-based midwife), and be visited postnatally by someone else, communications among the various providers are very important. Communications are facilitated by having the woman carry her own record, or part of it.

MATERNITY-RELATED BENEFITS

Every country provides paid maternity leave and sets protective limits on the working circumstances of pregnant women. Usual practice in most countries is to transfer women to nonstrenuous jobs as soon as pregnancy is confirmed. Night work for pregnant women is forbidden in the Netherlands, Belgium, Switzerland, and Federal Republic of Germany, although exceptions may be made in certain job categories or with the woman's consent. The law in several countries specifies that wages will continue during absences for prenatal visits or classes. The duration of maternity leave varies from a total of 9 weeks (Ireland) to 29 weeks (United Kingdom) (Table 7).

In most countries the leave is obligatory. In Switzerland, Norway, and Belgium the woman may elect to work until delivery and add the allowable prenatal leave to the postnatal leave. Similar postnatal extensions are permissible in the event of premature delivery. In Norway the father may take up to 12 weeks' paid postnatal leave if he is the principal care giver; the Federal Republic of Germany allows either parent to take postnatal leave.

The amount of pay during maternity leave varies from 100 percent of the mother's salary (usually to a maximum level) in Belgium, Federal Republic of Germany, Norway, and the Netherlands, to 90 percent of her salary in Denmark and France, and 75 percent in Spain. Ireland, the United Kingdom, and Switzerland provide a fixed payment, regardless of salary (EURO survey, 1982; Ierodiaconou, 1986).

The source of funds for paid maternity leave varies considerably. It is more often from social security or health insurance than directly from the employer, a circumstance that may protect against discrimination in the employment of women of childbearing age.

Leave can often be extended on an unpaid basis without loss of job or job-related benefits. Such extensions are possible in France and the Federal Republic of Germany for 1 to 3 years. In Belgium the period of unpaid

TABLE 7   Duration of Paid Maternity Leave in Study Countries,
1982, 1986

| Country | Leave (weeks) | |
	Prenatal	Postnatal
Belgium	6	8
Denmark	4	14[a]
Federal Republic of Germany	6	24
France	6	8
Ireland	6	3[a]
Netherlands	6	6
Norway	12	6
Spain[b]	6	8
Switzerland	8	8
United Kingdom	11	29

[a]Leave is extended for premature delivery.
[b]I. Alvarez, personal communication, 1987.

SOURCES: EURO survey, 1982; Ierodiaconou, E. 1986.

leave is extended to the end of the fifth month for mothers who breast-feed. All countries provide that additional paid sick leave may be given, if medically authorized. Payment during nursing breaks is ordinarily assured, ranging from two half-hour periods to two full-hour periods each day (France and Norway).

Maternity grants or bonuses, without means testing, are paid at the time of childbearing in all countries except Denmark. The payments are intended to assist with the cost of supplies and equipment for the new baby. Switzerland pays an additional bonus to mothers who breast-feed their babies. In all countries family allowances are paid for each child on a monthly basis, ordinarily until adulthood or completion of education. The amount of the monthly allowance varies with the number of children.

Some special maternity-related considerations are noteworthy. Belgium allows pregnant women first-class rail travel on a second-class ticket—a way of assuring a seat for pregnant women in a population of commuters. Additional considerations are given to single mothers in most countries. Priorities for day care and for public housing are well established for working mothers or for large families.

CONCLUSIONS

Review of pregnancy-related supports and services in 10 Western European countries with outstanding records of infant survival and low birthweight suggest that participation in early and continuous prenatal care can be achieved by:

- establishing easily understood and readily available provider systems;
- removing all barriers, especially economic ones, to the full range of services embraced by those systems; and
- linking prenatal care to comprehensive social and financial benefits that enable pregnant women and new mothers to protect their own well-being and to nurture their infants.

Inadequate scholarship exists to measure the relative importance of the several components of comprehensive perinatal care.

Most of the countries surveyed have established impressive programs of outreach featuring home visiting, which is designed primarily to prolong and enrich prenatal care rather than recruit women into care. Women appear to be attracted to prenatal care in order to avail themselves of the substantial medical and social benefits that attach to pregnancy and childbearing. Nothing in this analysis suggests that special endeavors or outreach in the absence of the above provisions will improve participation of pregnant women in prenatal care or improve outcomes of pregnancy.

REFERENCES

Blondel, B. 1987. Antenatal care in the European community countries over the last 20 years. In Perinatal Care Delivery Systems: Description and Evaluation in European Community Countries, M. Kaminski et al., eds. London: Oxford University Press.

Blondel, B., D. Pusch, and E. Schmidt. 1985. Some characteristics of antenatal care in 13 European countries. Brit. J. Obstet. Gynaecol. 9:565–568.

Buekens, P. 1987. Determinants of prenatal care. In Perinatal Care Delivery Systems: Description and Evaluation in European Community Countries, M. Kaminski et al., eds. London: Oxford University Press.

Children's Defense Fund. 1987. The Health of America's Children. Washington, D.C., p.7.

Demographic Yearbook. 1973 and 1983. New York: United Nations.

Doornbos, J. P. R., and H. J. Nordbeck. 1985. Perinatal Mortality. Obstetric Risk Factors in a Community of Mixed Ethnic Origin in Amsterdam. Amsterdam: B. V. Dordrecht.

Ierodiaconou, E. 1986. Maternity protection in 22 European countries. In Perinatal Health Services in Europe, J. M. L. Phaff, ed. Dover, N. H.: Croom Helm.

Institute of Medicine, 1985. Preventing Low Birthweight. Washington, D.C.: National Academy Press.

Jones, E. F., J. D. Forrest, N. Goldman, S. K. Henshaw, R. Lincoln, J. I. Rosoff, C. F. Westoff, and D. Wulf. 1985. Teenage pregnancy in developed countries: Determinants and policy implications. Fam. Plan. Perspect. 17:53–63.

Kaminiski, M., G. Breart, P. Buekens, H. J. Huisjes, G. McIlwaine, and H. K. Selbmann, eds. 1987. Perinatal Care Delivery Systems: Description and Evaluation in European Community Countries. London: Oxford University Press.

Kessner, D. M. 1973. Infant Death: An Analysis by Maternal Risk and Health Care. Washington, D.C.: Institute of Medicine.

Maxwell, J. 1984. Prenatal care and infant mortality: The French experience. Unpublished manuscript.

Miller, C. A., A. Fine, and S. Adams-Taylor. 1986. Monitoring Children's Health: Key Indicators. Washington, D.C.: American Public Health Association. .

National Center for Health Statistics. 1985a. Health United States, 1985. Hyattsville, Md.: U.S. Department of Health and Human Services.

National Center for Health Statistics. 1985b. Proceedings of the International Collaborative Effort on Perinatal and Infant Mortality, Vol. 1. Hyattsville, Md.: U.S. Department of Health and Human Services.

National Center for Health Statistics. 1987. Vital Statistics for the United States, 1985. Vol. 1, Natality. DHHS Publ. No. (PHS)87-1119. Washington, D.C.: Government Printing Office.

Notzon, F. C., P. J. Placek, and S. M. Taffel. 1987. Comparisons of National Cesarean Section Rates. N. Eng. J. Med. 316:386–389.

Phaff, J. M. L., ed. 1986. Perinatal Health Services in Europe. Dover, N. H.: Croom Helm.

Placek, P. J. 1986. Commentary: Caesarean rate still rising. Stat. Bull. 67(3):9.

Regional Office for Europe. 1985. Having a Baby in Europe. Copenhagen: World Health Organization.

Smedby, B., and A. Ericson. 1979. Perinatal mortality among children of immigrant women in Sweden. Acta Paedeatr. Scand. Suppl. 275(69):41–47.

UNICEF. 1987. The State of the World's Children 1987. Oxford: UNICEF.

Vandenbussche, P., E. Wollast, and P. Buekens. 1985. Some characteristics of antenatal care in 13 European countries. Brit. J. Obstet. Gynaecol. 92:1297.

Wallace, H. M. 1975. Health Care of Mothers and Children in National Health Services. Cambridge, Mass.: Ballinger.

World Bank. 1986. World Development Report. Oxford: World Bank.

World Health Organization. 1986. Evaluation of the Strategy for Health for All by the Year 2000, 7th Report on the World Health Situation. Vol. 5, European Regional Office. Copenhagen: WHO.

Appendix

C

The Medical Malpractice Crisis and Poor Women

Sara Rosenbaum and Dana Hughes

CAUSES OF THE INCREASE IN MALPRACTICE INSURANCE COSTS

In recent years, providers of obstetrical care have seen their malpractice insurance costs rise exponentially. A 1985 survey conducted by the American College of Obstetricians and Gynecologists (ACOG) found that more than 9 out of 10 members surveyed reported an increase in premiums during the previous 2 years, with the average increase equalling nearly $10,000. One in four physicians was confronted with an increase of $13,000 or more.[1] The mean malpractice premium expense paid in 1985 was $23,256—18 percent of a private obstetrician's total malpractice expenses and an increase of 28.8 percent more than 1982 prices.[2] Malpractice premium expenditures represent approximately 10 percent of an obstetrician's gross income.[3] By 1988, the average premium had risen to $37,015.[4]

The malpractice insurance crisis is part of a general explosion of liability insurance costs that has affected all sectors of society, from physicians to day care centers, bus companies, ice skating rinks, and vacation resorts. It began in 1974, when insurers began to escalate their rates[5] and has been part of an effort by insurers to limit their risks generally, whether in the area of liability or health or disability coverage.[6]

Sara Rosenbaum and Dana Hughes are Director, Health Division, and Senior Health Specialist, respectively, of the Children's Defense Fund, Washington, D.C.

There are several reasons why obstetrical malpractice costs have risen dramatically. These include medical advances, the demise of the locality rule, large awards, substandard physicians, contingency fees, the profit-seeking of insurance companies, and the underfinancing of maternity care.

Medical Advances and the Demise of the Locality Rule

Two simultaneous trends have had a major impact on obstetrical malpractice costs. The first is the extraordinary advances in the management of pregnancy and childbirth in the past two decades,[7] resulting in higher expectations regarding infant health. The second is the demise of the locality rule in tort litigation.[8]

Under the locality rule, an obstetrical defendant in a malpractice case could be held liable only if his or her care did not meet the professional standards of a reasonable obstetrician practicing within the defendant's local community. Over the past 20 years, however, the public, the judicial system, and insurers have begun to judge physicians by national standards. This is appropriate in a nation in which medical education takes place at nationally accredited medical schools and physicians are certified in specialties by national boards.[9] The demise of the locality rule has had two effects: it has brought national obstetrical standards into local communities, and it has made it far easier for medical experts from outside the local area to testify in malpractice trials.[10] Indeed, two noted experts have concluded that "the erosion of the 'locality rule' has probably had a greater impact on the increase in malpractice claims in recent years than any other change in the law."[11]

Large Awards

Another major cause of rising malpractice rates is the increase in the number of cases being filed and in the size of the awards being granted. Between 1976 and 1986, the number of insurance-related civil lawsuits doubled.[12] Between 1960 and 1980, the number of million-dollar judgments increased by more than 500 percent in some jurisdictions.[13] The average settlement grew from $5,000 in 1979 to $330,000 in 1986.[14]

As the number and size of claims have increased, insurers have experienced medical malpractice loss ratios (that is, combined loss and loss expenses over premium revenues) as much as 40 to 50 percent higher than the norm.[15] These high loss ratios have been intensified, according to insurers, by the long "tail" of malpractice cases—that is, the tendency of malpractice claims to be filed and resolved (either by settlement or litigation) anywhere from 5 to 13 years from the date of the incident.[16] High loss ratios and the so-called tail effect have also made it more difficult for insurance companies to find reinsurers that will accept malpractice risks.[17]

Substandard Physicians

A third probable cause of the increase in malpractice cases is the perception on the part of many persons that the medical profession does a poor job of policing itself and that malpractice litigation is the only mechanism for protecting against, and vindicating, wrongs that have been committed.[18] Anecdotes of physician abuses abound; indeed, James Todd of the American Medical Association recently stated that "the biggest cause of malpractice [litigation] is malpractice."[19] Not only do unhappy experiences with substandard practitioners fuel the malpractice fires, but very large awards in serious cases appear to have a greater effect on malpractice rates than do many small awards. Thus, the substandard performance of a handful of physicians can significantly affect the rate of all physicians in an area.[20]

Unfortunately, as will be discussed below, evidence suggests that malpractice litigation as a weapon is least available to those women and infants most likely to be furnished poor-quality medical care. Moreover, litigation is obviously no substitute for rigorous quality control, which is designed to prevent malpractice through such measures as specialized training, documented adherence to adequate practice protocols, and referrals to other care settings when necessary.

Contingency Fees

A fourth, and often discussed, cause of the malpractice crisis is lawyers' willingness to take on malpractice cases because of the potentially large awards, and correspondingly large contingency fees, involved. There is no question that the possibility of a large contingency fee is attractive; but it is likely that the demise of the locality rule has had a far greater impact on the growth of malpractice litigation, since medical malpractice cases turn on the ability to present expert testimony that a physician's conduct fell below professionally accepted standards.

Contingency fees have been severely criticized for promoting the filing of frivolous suits, yet between 50 and 75 percent of all malpractice claims brought to attorneys are refused, either because the merits of the claim or the size of the anticipated recovery would not justify the attorney's time and effort.[21] While contingency awards make it possible (and probably more attractive) to pursue claims, the Health Education and Welfare Secretary's Commission on Medical Malpractice found in 1973 that the "vast majority of malpractice claims are not entirely baseless."[22]

Insurance Companies

In addition to the demise of the locality rule, the most serious reason cited by some for the increase in malpractice rates is the profit seeking of insurance companies themselves. While premium payouts for malpractice claims have grown dramatically in recent years, there is evidence from the early days of the malpractice crisis that, contrary to being money losers, malpractice policies represent one of the most lucrative lines for the industry.[23] The financial rewards of malpractice insurance underwriting may be measured in several ways. First, while insurers cite the need for higher rates because of the tail effect in malpractice, that tail enables the industry to amass hundreds of millions of dollars in reserves that do not have to be paid out until many years into the future and that can be invested lucratively in the present. Thus, while malpractice policies themselves are not moneymakers, they represent a means of amassing large cash reserves.[24]

Second, the methodology used to project premium increases can yield tremendous profits for insurance companies because of its susceptibility to manipulation. Establishing a premium rate is a function of (1) the number of *exposures to claims* a physician or medical group will generate in a year (an occurrence estimate); (2) the anticipated number of losses those exposures will yield; and (3) the rate and dollar amount by which claims will increase or decrease in a year.[25] At each stage, insurance companies can overstate the situation, thereby projecting a highly inflated claims and cost profile. Few insurance commissions carefully scrutinize these projections; when they do, rate increases are frequently denied.[26]

Third, with the transition from individual to group policy underwriting that occurred by the mid-1970s, the probability of price gouging and monopolistic practices heightened. It is no coincidence, in the view of some experts, that the malpractice crisis occurred simultaneously with the elimination of all but a few insurers from the malpractice underwriting business.[27]

Underfinancing of Maternity Care

Finally, the gross underfinancing of obstetrical care in the United States may itself be propelling malpractice claims. More than 14 million American women are uninsured for maternity care, and two-thirds of these— over 9 million persons—are without any health insurance whatever.[28] Physicians faced with the management of inadequately financed patients may be unable to provide or arrange for optimal care. In at least one instance, a Medicaid agency has been unsuccessfully sued over its failure to approve payments for procedures that the beneficiary's physicians deemed medically essential.[29]

Much attention has been paid to the impact of defensive medicine on medical inflation; less has been paid to the impact of underfunding on the medical community's ability to furnish appropriate care. For example, no single component of maternity care is more crucial to a good birth outcome than delivery in a setting appropriate to the risk involved in the pregnancy. According to experts, women at high risk of adverse outcomes of pregnancy should be delivered in inpatient hospitals with appropriately advanced neonatal care facilities. Yet a recent national survey of state-funded maternity programs for uninsured low-income women found that fewer than half the programs covered inpatient delivery services at all.[30] Women in states that do not cover delivery costs are expected to make their own financial arrangements for admission. This means that they are dependent upon hospitals that will admit them free of charge or at least without a sizable preadmission deposit, regardless of whether their physicians have admitting privileges there or whether the hospital is equipped to meet their medical needs. Indeed, one state health official responded flatly that the regionalized perinatal system in her state was only available to insured women.[31] As a result, proper management of high-risk maternity cases involving uninsured women may be virtually impossible in half the states.

Response by Providers of Obstetrical Care

Whatever the causes of the malpractice crisis, it has elicited several responses from the obstetrical community, all of which affect the poor most severely. First, large numbers of providers have simply ceased furnishing obstetrical care. Second, public health providers' ability to obtain insurance coverage has been threatened, leading to the reduction or elimination of subsidized maternity care. Third, many obstetricians have begun to reject high-risk cases, which they perceive as occurring disproportionately among poor and difficult patients, in order to avoid future liability. Finally, the crisis has caused many providers of obstetrical care to reject underfinanced (or completely unfinanced) persons who cannot pay their way.

Cessation of Obstetrical Practice

Studies indicated that, particularly in states with excessively high malpractice rates, physicians have ceased furnishing obstetrical care entirely. A 1988 ACOG survey of professional liability revealed that 12.4

percent of all responding obstetricians and 25.1 percent of Florida respondents have given up the practice of obstetrics altogether.[32] Twenty-five percent of California obstetricians responding to a survey reported that they had completely ceased furnishing deliveries.[33] Community Health Center directors in Florida, Texas, California, and New York report that private obstetricians who used to take referrals no longer do so because they have given up obstetrical practice. In some communities, particularly those with poorer populations and no teaching or public facilities, obstetrical care may simply be disappearing.

Impact on Providers of Maternity Care to the Poor

One of the most grievous effects of the malpractice crisis has been its impact on providers that represent the major source of obstetrical care for poor women, such as Title V-funded health clinics, Community and Migrant Health Centers, public hospitals and clinics, and nurse–midwife practices. Public and quasi-public clinics are modestly funded and cannot afford monumentally costly insurance policies, nor can nurse–midwives, with their average annual salary of $25,000. Yet even though both Community Health Centers and nurse–midwives have very low malpractice claims profiles compared to other providers of obstetrical care, their rates have risen dramatically.[34]

Health centers' rates have skyrocketed so high that centers are shutting down obstetrical programs. According to the National Association of Community Health Centers, policies that cost between $800 and $900 in 1985 cost $12,000 in 1986.[35] In one graphic example, the Anchorage Neighborhood Health Center in Alaska, which performed 300 deliveries in 1985 and was expected to perform 500 in 1986, was told that the malpractice premium for its six obstetricians in 1986 would rise from $40,000 to between $200,000 and $400,000. As a result, the center eliminated four of its six obstetricians and dropped the number of deliveries from 500 to 150.[36] The remaining women presumably either went without care or else relied on whatever charitable services they could locate. Numerous centers report that, while their staff continue to provide prenatal care, the malpractice crisis has forced them to cease providing delivery services because the additional premium cost they would incur in order to insure their physicians is far too high. For example, at one center in Florida, malpractice coverage for prenatal care services is $4,000 annually per staff member. Coverage for delivery, however, would add $25,000 in costs per staff person. Physicians at the center thus are faced with "going bare" and delivering their patients without coverage, or effectively abandoning their patients at the time of delivery, which ironically, could easily lead to malpractice litigation.

Rejection of High-Risk Women

According to the 1988 ACOG survey, rising malpractice rates have led more than 27 percent of all responding obstetricians to reduce their high-risk caseloads.[37] A separate survey of California obstetricians found that nearly 50 percent reported reducing their high-risk caseloads.[38] This desire to avoid cases that pose high medical risks undoubtedly has led many obstetricians to stop treating publicly insured and uninsured low-income pregnant women on the premise that they are medically at risk.

However, even if one assumes that high-risk cases are more common among low-income women, rejecting such patients may have little or no bearing on the number of malpractice claims filed against a physician. To understand why this is so, it is important to understand how medical malpractice policies are written. A malpractice policy is written on an occurrence basis; that is, an insured physician is covered for all *claims* arising from incidents (*not* for any incidents of malpractice that actually might arise) that occur in the year for which the policy is written.[39] Thus, the key is really *whether an incident leads to a claim*, not simply whether an incident actually occurs. Actuaries project how many incidents will eventually result in claims; thus the skills and conduct of the physician may be significantly less important than the likelihood that a particular group of patients will sue.

While an in-depth analysis of claims filed is needed to determine who is likely to sue, the modest evidence that already exists suggests that, regardless of whether poor women are more likely to be at risk or to suffer from actual incidents of malpractice, they are less likely than nonpoor women to present claims. Lower-income persons were significantly less likely to have ever reported any incident and one-half as likely to have reported two or more incidents. Similarly, persons with little education were only about half as likely to report any incident and one-third as likely to report one, two, or more incidents.

A malpractice study conducted by the National Association of Community Health Centers in 1986 showed that center obstetricians (virtually all of whose patients have incomes that are less than 200 percent of the federal poverty level, and 25 to 40 percent of whom are eligible for Medicaid)[40] have malpractice claim profiles approximately one-fifth as great as that of office-based obstetricians, who, even several years ago, were the least likely of all primary care physicians to accept any Medicaid patients in their practices.[41]

A recent General Accounting Office (GAO) study of the characteristics of medical malpractice claims closed in 1984 sheds some additional light on the issue of who files claims.[42] Unfortunately, the study provides financial information only on patient earnings, as opposed to total family income, and only in the aggregate, not for specific subpopulations. (Children represented 17 percent of all claims closed in 1984, and one-third of those claims involved allegations of obstetrical malpractice.)

The GAO study does, however, report the source of patients' health care financing prior to the incident on which the claim was based, which allows one to infer their general economic status at that time. It also allows one to differentiate between persons who became eligible for public medical assistance only after the occurrence of a disabling incident and persons who were poor enough to qualify for public medical assistance beforehand.

Of all claims closed in 1984, only 3.9 percent of claimants were Medicaid patients at the time of their injuries. This number is disproportionately low in relation to Medicaid representation in the population at large, suggesting that Medicaid patients (and thus poor persons) are less likely to file claims. Thus, while the GAO insurance data are not reported by age or sex and are limited only to a sample of claims closed in 1984 by 25 insurers, they do tend to confirm earlier studies suggesting that the poor are less, rather than more, likely to sue.

Finally, a recent study conducted for ACOG found that women covered by Medicaid for their hospital delivery were somewhat more likely than other women to file a malpractice claim against the hospital, but this finding was not statistically significant.[43] The study suffers from substantial flaws, however.

First, the researchers' identifications of claimants were based on the payer of delivery costs. In thousands of cases, Medicaid pays retroactively for delivery costs incurred by women who were ineligible for coverage during their pregnancies and at the time of delivery as well. This retroactive feature seriously compromises any effort to discern malpractice claims patterns among Medicaid-financed women. Many women ostensibly insured by Medicaid were in fact completely uninsured for both prenatal care and delivery services; only much later were they found eligible for Medicaid.

Second, the study measures claims against hospitals rather than claims against physicians. A disproportionate number of Medicaid-insured and uninsured women depend on hospital staff (that is, interns and residents) for both medical and hospital care; thus, even if they did file claims with any greater frequency than other types of patients, it might have little or no bearing on their behavior toward office-based physicians.

Third, the findings were based on all claims made against the responding hospitals, including claims that were later dropped. Because of the great difficulties that Medicaid beneficiaries and other poor persons face in obtaining legal assistance, the number of claims generated by Medicaid patients may be significantly overrepresentative of all claims that are ultimately paid.

Finally, the report sheds no light on the size of the claim nor the incident that forms that basis of the complaint. As a result, there is no means of separating out either high-impact claims (since it is the very large claims that affect physicians' malpractice premium rates most) or meritorious claims.

Why fewer malpractice claims appear to arise from poor women probably has less to do with the quality of care they receive than with their failure to understand that potential malpractice has been committed, their fears about pressing their claims, and their inability to secure legal assistance. Indeed, except for communities served by Community Health Centers, specialized clinical or hospital-based perinatal projects, or other public providers, poor women and their infants probably face a greater risk than any other group of women and children of receiving substandard care from either nonspecialty physicians or relatively untrained interns and residents. The heightened risk can be seen in the elevated maternal and infant mortality rates that plague the low-income population. A significant amount of this mortality has been deemed preventable by experts.

It is evident that, even among the general population, there is only a small likelihood that an injured person will file a claim. The Commission on Medicaid Malpractice found that, while 7.5 percent of all hospital discharges involved an iatrogenic injury and 30 percent of them were caused by negligence, only 1.7 percent resulted in a claim and only one-third of that number obtained a recovery.[44] Another study found that only 10 percent of injured persons file a claim and only 4 percent achieve a recovery.[45]

Poor women may be even less likely to sue. They have less contact with the health system generally, and when they do it is more likely to be within a relatively forbidding institutional setting in which they feel powerless, as opposed to a one-on-one, empowering, ongoing relationship with a single physician. Because the poor traditionally have received less and poorer-quality medical care, they may be less aware of what a positive medical experience should be and less inclined to take action against even gross malpractice.

When poor women do wish to act on an incident, they confront enormous barriers to finding an attorney. First, legal services attorneys may not accept malpractice cases unless no pro bono assistance is available or the claimant has been denied even a consultation—not actual representation—by two attorneys.[46] Attorneys refuse nearly three-quarters of the malpractice claims brought to them, whether because the claim is without merit, the case is too difficult to prove, the recovery amount is too small to be worth their time, or there exist legal defenses to the providers' actions.

Private lawyers may be even more likely to reject poor women's claims. The way medical malpractice recoveries are valued reduces the size of the award an attorney can anticipate, and special defenses are often available to institutions serving the poor.

Attorneys freely admit that the amount of the economic loss claimed is a major factor in deciding whether to take a case.[47] Economic loss is chiefly a function of out-of-pocket costs, lost earning capacity, and pain and suffering. As limits are placed on pain and suffering awards (see the discussion below) and as more state legislatures overturn the so-called collateral source rule (which prohibits malpractice defendants from presenting evidence that plaintiffs can collect for their injuries from other sources, such as insurance, Supplemental Security Income, and Medicaid), the lost earnings factor becomes increasingly important.

In the case of poor persons, estimates of lost earning capacity are set low.[48] Moreover, when poor women or children who are also Medicaid recipients do recover a major award, the law's third-party liability and liens and recoveries provisions require that they turn over their awards to the state, to the extent that the state pays for care.[49] While courts have ruled that attorneys do have the right to recover their fees in these situations, at least one state has determined that attorneys are not entitled to collect any part of their fee from the proceeds due the state for medical assistance rendered.[50] This reduces considerably the size of the award on which an attorney's fee will be based. In short, the Medicaid provisions make it less in the interest of recipients to file claims and less in the interest of attorneys to bring them.

Certain defenses are available to defendants serving large numbers of poor patients that may not be available to other providers. For example, public providers may be protected from suit by sovereign immunity. Nonprofit providers are protected in some jurisdictions by the common law (or statutory) doctrine of charitable immunity.[51] And physicians who perform deliveries in emergencies are frequently provided a good Samaritan defense, so long as they have not been grossly negligent and have not had reasonable access to the women's medical records.[52]

In sum, there is certainly evidence that poor women pose higher medical risks than nonpoor women insofar as obstetrical care and pregnancy outcomes are concerned. But higher risk in and of itself does not affect a physician's malpractice exposure *if the incidents do not become claims*. The health profiles of poor women often dictate more intensive care, but evidence suggests that poor women are less likely to sue. While no definitive measures can be provided without an audit of all claims filed against obstetrical providers, the evidence on malpractice litigants points away from the poor.

Rejection of Underfinanced Women

One clear response to the malpractice crisis has been a widespread refusal among obstetrical providers to see publicly insured and uninsured persons. As previously noted, a preponderance of obstetricians and gynecologists has traditionally refused to treat Medicaid patients, but over the past several years news stories from around the nation have reported a wholesale pullout by obstetricians from Medicaid and other public health programs in many communities.[53] In each instance, low reimbursement rates are cited as the main reason. A recent analysis by the Texas Health Department of implementation of the 1985 Maternity and Infant Health Improvement Act reported as follows:

> The most severe issue to face the program is that of malpractice insurance of health providers. Many physicians, in particular those practicing in obstetrics, have been deterred from participating in the program because of concerns about increased liability, about alleged increases in their own malpractice insurance premiums and in some instances, about the inability to obtain any malpractice insurance at all if they accept indigent high risk women as patients. . . . Some hospitals have expressed the same reasons but are also very concerned about what they see as the very low reimbursement offered. . . .[54]

As reimbursement rates fall behind the per-capita cost of practice (which includes the per patient cost of malpractice premiums), physicians are increasingly unwilling to shift costs to make up for the losses they suffer from treating publicly insured and uninsured women, particularly given their general unwillingness to treat such women to begin with.

STATE RESPONSES

The states' responses to the malpractice crisis as of 1986 commonly include:[55]

- Elimination of the collateral source rule, including express legislation that classifies as a collateral source medical and disability payments by the Social Security Administration and other federal, state, and local public aid programs.
- Limitations on recoveries for noneconomic damage.
- Curbs on the filing of frivolous claims.
- Elimination of the joint and several liability rule, which makes defendants liable for damages in excess of their actual liability if other defendants are unable to pay.
- Limitations on contingency fees.
- Mandatory cooling off periods prior to the filing of a claim.
- Staff discipline measures, including, in one state, a requirement that all obstetrical physicians perform risk assessments and refer patients to appropriate facilities as a condition of insurance coverage.
- Establishment of prelitigation arbitration panels.

- Joint underwriting associations (JUAs), which underwrite malpractice insurance for providers unable to secure coverage from another source.
- Shortened statutes of limitations, particularly in the case of injuries to minors, in order to reduce the tail effect.
- Establishment of patient compensation funds.
- Increases in Medicaid payment rates to better enable providers to cover their costs.
- Periodic payment rules to guard against sudden windfall outlays.

If the demise of the locality rule and the move by insurers to build up large reserves against what they estimate to be major risks truly lie at the heart of the malpractice crisis, then the above state actions may produce very little relief. Indeed, a recent study by GAO concludes that very few reforms have had a major impact.[56]

No policymakers appear to have suggested resuscitating the locality rule, since there is widespread belief among physicians, insurers, and consumers that, at least in certain medical disciplines, national standards of practice can, and must, be articulated. Interest groups are split as to whether the best solution is to raise the standards by which fault is established or substitute a no-fault resolution mechanism in place of the current system.[57]

Conclusion and Recommendations

The basic issue of whether to modify the fault system or switch to a no-fault system is one for long-term debate. In the interim, several things might be done to protect poor women:

- States might use their JUAs to set up a subsidized, umbrella malpractice plan for all physicians who practice at, or accept referrals from, public, hospital-based, and other clinics for the poor. Physicians who furnish prenatal care in their offices might also be brought under the umbrella. States might abandon a risk model altogether in the case of obstetrics and establish no-fault compensation systems. In 1987, Virginia enacted legislation to establish a program to compensate patients suffering birth-related neurological injuries. This program will be available to physicians and hospitals who agree to provide obstetrical care for Medicaid recipients and indigent patients, pay an annual fee, and submit to a review of all claims by the Board of Medicine. The fee ($5,000 in the case of physicians) is subsidized by an annual levy of $250 on nonparticipating physicians. Hospitals must pay $50 per delivery.
- States should raise reimbursement rates for obstetrical care under Medicaid and indigent health insurance to better cover the cost of malpractice insurance.

• States should watch more carefully the process of setting malpractice insurance rates. Insurance companies' projections of the likelihood of litigation—particularly their tendency to use projections from high-litigation states in low-litigation jurisdictions—merit scrutiny.

References and Notes

1. American College of Obstetricians and Gynecologists, *Professional Liability Insurance and Its Effects* (Washington, D.C., 1985).
2. Adams, E. Kathleen, and Burfield, W. Bradley, "Malpractice Premium Expenses: Another 'Crisis' and Its Implications," *Medical Benefits* (Kelley Communications, Charlottesville, Va.), April 15, 1988, p. 6.
3. ACOG, *op. cit.*
4. American College of Obstetricians and Gynecologists, *Professional Liability and Its Effects: Report of a 1987 Survey of ACOG's Membership* (Washington, D.C., 1988).
5. Law, Sylvia, and Polan, Steven, *Pain and Profit: The Politics of Malpractice* (New York: Harper & Row, 1978).
6. Just as insurers have sought to limit their exposure to liability awards by refusing to cover certain classes of activities or by extending coverage only at prohibitive rates, they have also sought to limit their exposure in other areas. For example, companies that now underwrite group medical insurance plans routinely attach riders prohibiting coverage for preexisting conditions or for certain diagnoses (such as AIDS or cancer). Thus, insurers' behavior in malpractice coverage parallels their behavior in other areas of risk taking. See Rosenbaum, Sara, "Children and Private Health Insurance," in *Children in a Changing Health Care System*, Schlesinger, Marle, ed. (Baltimore: Johns Hopkins University Press, in press).
7. Institute of Medicine, *Preventing Low Birthweight* (Washington, D.C.: National Academy Press, 1986).
8. Law and Polan, *op. cit.*, p. 100.
9. *Ibid.*
10. Finding expert witnesses from the defendant's community who were willing to testify has traditionally been one of the greatest barriers to malpractice cases.
11. Law and Polan, *op. cit.*, pp. 1–8.
12. Nicholas, Nancy, "The Manufacturing of a Crisis," *The Nation*, February 15, 1986, pp. 173–175.
13. *Ibid.*
14. Intergovernmental Health Policy Project, *State Health Notes* (Washington, D.C.: George Washington University, 1987), p. 1.
15. "Reforming Malpractice Law," *Washington Report on Medicine and Health* (George Washington University) September 30, 1985, p. 1.
16. ACOG, *op. cit.*, 1985, p. 4.
17. "Reforming Malpractice," *op. cit.*, p. 2.
18. Indeed, the report of the HEW Secretary's Commission on Medical Malpractice of 1973 found that attitudes toward physicians and the desire to indicate a perceived harm lay at the heart of many malpractice claims.
19. Quoted in *Health Advocate* (National Health Law Program, Los Angeles), Spring 1986, p. 3.
20. Law and Polan, *op. cit.* The authors note that, according to the National Association of Insurance Commissioners, in 1975 claims of $50,000 or more

accounted for only 3 percent of claims made but 63 percent of premiums paid out. Thus the large claims tend to drive payout rates.

21. *Ibid.*
22. Cited in Law and Polan, *op. cit.*, pp. 28–50.
23. Law and Polan, *op. cit.*, p. 161.
24. *Ibid.*, pp. 161–194; Nichols, *op. cit.*, p. 3.
25. Law and Polan, *op. cit.*, p. 178.
26. *Ibid.*
27. *Ibid.*
28. Alan Guttmacher Institute, *Blessed Events and the Bottom Line* (New York, 1988).
29. *Wickline* v. *State of California*, No. 13010156 (California Court of Appeal, July 30, 1986). Reprinted in CCA *Medicare/Medicaid Guide*, par. 36,325.
30. Rosenbaum, Sara, Hughes, Dana, and Johnson, Kay, "Maternal and Child Health Services for Medically Indigent Children and Pregnant Women," *Medical Care* 26 (1988):315–332.
31. *Ibid.*
32. ACOG, *op. cit.*, 1988, p. 22.
33. Survey reported in "Reforming Malpractice," *op. cit.*, p. 2.
34. A 1986 study of the medical malpractice claims experience of Community and Migrant Health Centers conducted by the National Association of Community Health Centers in Washington, D.C., revealed that, while 75 percent of all private obstetrics/gynecology specialists had at least one claim filed against them in 1985, only 16 percent of such specialists practicing at Community and Migrant Health Centers had a claim filed. Similarly, because only 6 percent of all nurse–midwives have had claims filed, their rates should be modest; yet in 1985 midwives lost their coverage entirely.
35. National Association of Community Health Centers, "Medical Malpractice: Here We Go Again," *NACH Newsletter*, Winter, 1986, pp. 1–4.
36. *Ibid.*, p. 3.
37. ACOG, *op. cit.*, 1988, p. 22.
38. "Reforming Malpractice," *op. cit.*, p. 3.
39. Law and Polan, *op. cit.*, pp. 97–116.
40. Rosenbaum, Sara, *Two Decades of Achievement* (Washington, D.C.: National Association of Community Health Centers, 1986).
41. Mitchell, Janet, and Cromwell, Jerry, "Medicaid Mills: Fact or Fiction?" *Health Care Financing Review*, Summer 1980, pp. 1–33. The authors report that, while 21.6 percent of all primary care physicians refused any Medicaid patients in their practices, 36.8 percent of obstetricians/gynecologists saw no such patients. Moreover, the latter were only about two-thirds as likely as primary care physicians to have a large Medicaid practice.
42. U.S. General Accounting Office, *Medical Malpractice; Characteristics of Claims Closed in 1984*, GAO-HRD-87-55 (Washington, D.C.: Government Printing Office, 1987).
43. Opinion Research Corporation, *Hospital Survey on Obstetric Claim Frequency* (Washington, D.C., 1988).
44. *Health Advocate*, February 1986, p. 3.
45. *Ibid.*, p. 3.
46. *Ibid.*, p. 2.
47. Law and Polan, *op. cit.*
48. *Ibid.*
49. 42 U.S.C. par. 1396a(a)(18)(a)(25).

50. Attorney General op., New York, March 20, 1981.
51. See, e.g., *Ponder et al.* v. *Fulton-DeKalb Hospital Authority* Georgia Civil Action, 1986.
52. See, e.g., legislation enacted by Virginia in 1987 that provides as follows:

    Any person who, in the absence of gross negligence, renders emergency obstetrical care or assistance to a female in active labor who has not previously been cared for in connection with the pregnancy by such person or by another professionally associated with such person and whose medical records are not reasonably available to such person shall not be liable for any civil damages for acts or omissions resulting from the rendering of such emergency care or assistance. The immunity herein granted shall apply only to the emergency medical care provided.

53. Stories have appeared in newspapers in Massachusetts, Rhode Island, Maryland, California, New York, and Florida, to name only some.
54. *Indigent Care Programs: Annual Report* (Austin: Texas Department of Health, 1987).
55. See, generally, Intergovernmental Health Policy Project, *State Health Notes* (September 1986).
56. U.S. General Accounting Office, *Medical Malpractice: No Agreement on the Problems or Solutions*, GAO-HRD-86-50 (Washington, D.C.: Government Printing Office, 1986).
57. *Ibid.*

Index

245